CyberKnife Radiosurgery
A Practical Guide

Editor
M. Peter Heilbrun

The CyberKnife Society
1310 Chesapeake Terrace
Sunnyvale CA 94089

CyberKnife Radiosurgery: A Practical Guide

Copyright © 2003 by The CyberKnife Society

All rights reserved. No part of this book shall be reproduced, stored in a retrieval system, or transmitted in any means, electronic, mechanical, photocopying, recording, or otherwise, without written permission from the publisher. No patent liability is assumed with respect to the use of the information contained herein. Although every precaution has been taken in the preparation of this book, the publisher and authors assume no responsibility for errors or omissions. Neither is liability assumed for damages resulting from the use of information contained herein.

International Standard Book Number - 0-9753124-0-5

Library of Congress Control Number - 2004103876

Printed in the United States of America

Third Printing: March 2005

Trademarks

All terms mentioned in this book that are known to be trademarks or service marks have been appropriately capitalized. The editors cannot attest to the accuracy of this information. Use of a term in this Book should not be regarded as affecting the validity of any trademark or service mark.

Warning and Disclaimer

Every effort has been made to make this book as complete and accurate as possible, but no warranty of fitness is implied. The information provided by the editor and contributors is on an "as is" basis. The editors and publisher shall have neither liability or responsibility to any person or entity with respect to any loss or damages arising from the information contained in this book or accompanying electronic data.

Publisher

The CyberKnife Society
1310 Chesapeake Terrace
Sunnyvale CA 94089

List of Contributors

John R. Adler Jr., M.D.
Professor of Neurosurgery
Department of Neurosurgery
Stanford University Medical Center

Steven D. Chang, M.D.
Assistant Professor of Neurosurgery
Department of Neurosurgery
Stanford University Medical Center

Peter C. Gerszten, M.D., MPH
Assistant Professor of Neurosurgery
Department of Neurological Surgery
University of Pittsburgh School of Medicine

Iris C. Gibbs, M.D.
Assistant Professor of Radiation Oncology
Department of Radiation Oncology
Stanford University Medical Center

M. Peter Heilbrun, M.D.
Professor of Neurosurgery
Department of Neurosurgery
Stanford University Medical Center

Gary Heit, M.D., Ph.D.
Assistant Professor of Neurosurgery
Department of Neurosurgery
Stanford University Medical Center

Anthony Ho, Ph.D.
Medical Physicist
Department of Radiation Oncology
Stanford University Medical Center

Laurence Jang, R.T.T.
Radiation Therapist
Department of Radiation Oncology
Stanford University Medical Center

Martin Murphy, Ph.D.
Associate Professor of Radiation Oncology
Virginia Commonwealth University
Medical College of Virginia

Derek Olender
Clinical Education Specialist
Accuray Inc.

Pantaleo Romanelli, M.D.
Instructor in Neurosurgery
Department of Neurosurgery
Stanford University Medical Center

William C. Welch, M.D.
Assistant Professor of Neurosurgery
Department of Neurological Surgery
University of Pittsburgh School of Medicine

Table of Contents

Foreword vi

Introduction and Overview 8

Cranial Radiosurgery 10

CyberKnife Radiosurgery for the Spine 20

CyberKnife Radiosurgery for Trigeminal Neuralgia 32

Radiobiology and Radiosurgery 38

CyberKnife Image Guidance and Tracking 44

CyberKnife Physics and Quality Assurance 50

The Treatment Planning System 62

CyberKnife Setup and Treatment 76

Fiducials for Target Localization 80

Foreword

M. Peter Heilbrun

The CyberKnife radiosurgery system has the unique capability of non-isocentric beam delivery, thus allowing a highly conformal radiation dose to a target volume with a steep dose gradient that minimizes radiation to surrounding structures. At the same time, near real time image guidance allows the tracking of target movement. These two unique CyberKnife processes of non-isocentric beam delivery and image guidance are major technical advances in radiation delivery.

The goal of this guide is to provide an easy to use starting point for physicians, therapists, and physicists to familiarize themselves with the present state of CyberKnife radiosurgery. I have no doubt that new users will incorporate their own expertise in ways that the authors of this guide may not have considered. I have asked my colleagues at Stanford, University of Pittsburgh, and Accuray to contribute to this guide knowing that by the time it is published, many new ideas and uses will have evolved.

Radiosurgery evolution--an overview of the early systems and their limitations. Early standard linear accelerator and cobalt-60 (Gamma Knife) radiosurgery systems delivered a single, relatively spherical dose of focused radiation to a treatment volume by firing a collection of radiation beams arranged around a sphere. The dose gradients, displayed for planning as a series of isodose values in overlapping shells, showed the distribution and volume of radiation doses to normal tissues that surround a target volume. However, when target volumes were not spherical, using a single cylindrical beam collimator to deliver an encompassing lethal dose also delivered a lethal dose to portions of surrounding normal tissue.

The first effort to decrease the adjacent tissue dose used multiple iso-center treatment methods to define multiple target points within a target volume. This technique achieved not only a more conformal radiation dose to the target volume, but also a reduced dose to the surrounding normal tissue. Nevertheless, there are disadvantages to multiple iso-center treatment planning and delivery methods. For example, increased treatment time occurs because each iso-center must be at the focal point of the linear accelerator or the cobalt-60 radiosurgery systems. Therefore, the patient, wearing a stereotactic frame, must be physically moved within the confines of the center of the radiation treatment space. Additionally, while multiple iso-center plans are designed to minimize dose to normal structures, they often result in areas of higher or lower than desired radiation (hot spots and cold spots) both within and outside the boundary of a target volume.

In standard linear accelerator systems, the adaptation of multi-leaf collimators (MLC's) to shape the radiation beam was the next major advance to improve the homogeneity and conformality of a target volume dose. Both static and dynamic multi-leaf collimators can conform to the two-dimensional profile or shape of a three-dimensional target volume along the orthogonal or 90 degree axis of a specific beam trajectory. Generally, MLC's are used in a single iso-center method which eliminates the complexities and problems of multiple iso-center treatment. Although cobalt-60 systems cannot use MLC's for beam shaping, the conformality of treatments may be increased by 1) using small collimators, 2) blocking beam apertures, and 3) treating the target volume border to the 50% isodose, which is the steepest part of the dose gradient curve.

All methods of delivering conformal doses of radiation reduce the radiation dose to surrounding normal tissue. However, because the standard linac can only adjust the beam position utilizing two degrees of rotation, i.e., the vertical rotation of the linac gantry in one plane around the target focal point, and the horizontal rotation of the linac table holding the patient, the possibilities for beam selection and weighting are limited. Likewise, with cobalt-60 radiosurgery systems, once the target volume is moved along a single horizontal axis into the head vault, there are no degrees of movement and the beam selection depends on apertures holding the 201 cobalt sources.

Also, the radiation dose varies based on the distance from the radiation source to the target and the passage through air and tissue. With both the standard linac and the cobalt-60 systems, the source to target distance is fixed. Finally, radiosurgical target volumes traditionally have been small, averaging about 3 cubic centimeters. When target volumes exceed 20 cubic centimeters, conformal doses may not reduce significantly the dose to surrounding tissues. In this situation, many radio-surgeons and radiation oncologists recommend static conformal IMRT with standard dose division or fractionation regimens, rather than single stage radiosurgical treatment.

The CyberKnife solution. John Adler's imaginative invention, which mates a lightweight linear accelerator designed to inspect missile silos and other large structures to a six degrees of freedom robot, makes target planning more precise and eliminates the need for rigid restraints. Additionally, because of the precision and ease of the CyberKnife's frameless tracking, many users have instituted protocols for staged CyberKnife treatments of larger tumor volumes. Thus, the CyberKnife's ability to use a robotic manipulator to guide a set of radiation beams to any point within a target volume, combined with its radiographic and optical guidance systems, has revolutionized the field of radiosurgery.

The decade of the 1990's led to manufacture of the first CyberKnife prototypes tested at Stanford and several other sites in the United States and Japan. The system received FDA clearance to market the device to treat lesions of the head, neck, and upper spine in 1999. FDA market clearance for treatment of lesions anywhere in the body where radiation therapy is used was granted in late 2001. Since then, there has been a steady increase in installations of CyberKnife systems in visionary academic and community medical institutions in the USA, Asia, and Europe.

Again, this guide is a start. Nevertheless, I hope it is helpful for both neophyte and experienced proponents of focused radiation techniques for the management of human disease.

I would like to acknowledge my colleagues at Stanford, the University of Pittsburgh, and Accuray for their timely contributions. I thank David Martin, M.D. for introducing me to the power and subtleties of the CyberKnife treatment planning software. I also thank the staff at Accuray for their support for the CyberKnife Society. Last and not least, I thank my wife, Robyn.

M. Peter Heilbrun, M.D.

Introduction and Overview

John R. Adler, Jr.

Serendipity alone sent me to the Karolinska Institute in 1985 on a one year neurosurgical fellowship. Once there, I quickly fell under the spell of Professor Lars Leksell. Although previously trained at Harvard by some of the best American neurosurgeons, I was truly awed by the clinical results that Leksell's team was achieving with the Gamma Knife for a broad range of brain disorders. Yes, radiosurgery lacked the drama of open neurosurgery. However, the clinical advantages for selected patients seemed unarguable. That one small insight, and the sheer luck through which I repeatedly ended up at the right place at the right time, has enabled the evolution of the CyberKnife as it exists today.

As conceived by Leksell, there are two elemental principles of radiosurgery. The first is that, if a brain lesion can be imaged, it can be accurately targeted through the principles of stereotactic localization. The second is that by utilizing the concept of cross-fired beams to administer ablative doses of high-energy radiation, one can destroy the targeted brain lesion without injuring the surrounding normal tissue. Needless to say, the field of radiosurgery has since become much more complex as a range of new technologies has evolved. However, Leksell's basic radiosurgical tenets remain essentially invariant. Despite the obvious power of Leksell's vision, its shortcomings were also readily apparent. The greatest limitation stemmed from the absolute need to use stereotactic frames for radiosurgical targeting. The specific problems posed by the frame included:

1) limited ability to fractionate larger tumors and lesions next to radiosensitive critical structures, 2) mechanical limitations precluding treatment of lesions at the extremes of the brain, and 3) no ability, and no potential, to treat targets outside the head. The last of the above shortcomings is particularly important, since the vast majority of solid tumors occur outside the brain. Ultimately, these limitations provided the impetus for a completely new approach to radiosurgery, which eventually evolved into the modern CyberKnife.

CyberKnife Overview

The CyberKnife combines a number of advanced technologies and is by any measure a complex instrument to use. Its complexity stems directly from the need for maximal system flexibility. Furthermore, the entire field of extracranial radiosurgery is in its infancy, and therefore the treatment of many anatomic targets is far from streamlined. This complexity, and the lack of mature processes, makes thorough training an issue of paramount importance. This manual is intended to address this need.

It cannot be emphasized enough that the clinical application of radiosurgery to many extracranial lesions is still very much a work-in-progress. That does not mean that such treatment is ineffective. Actually it is quite the contrary, since the preliminary clinical outcome after CyberKnife treatment of extracranial tumors has been uniformly excellent. But such results should not be surprising, given the huge prior experience with treating biologically similar intracranial lesions with all forms of radiosurgery. However, as our experience has grown, so has our capacity to improve significantly upon initial procedures. Undoubtedly, a rewriting of this monograph would look very different even 2 years from now, and I thoroughly expect today's student, to be tomorrow's teacher.

Like other stereotactic brain procedures, and, for that matter, almost all of surgery, to be successful, CyberKnife radiosurgery requires exquisite attention to detail. Moreover, even though CyberKnife procedures will become ever more automated over time, the safe use of this instrument will always demand attentive skilled human oversight. Machines will just about always do what they are instructed, even when such instructions are inherently dangerous. Therefore, the CyberKnife must be operated by a team of skilled physicians and physicist/technicians, all of whom can provide checks on the decisions of each other. Successful operation of the CyberKnife requires teamwork, on-the-fly decision-making, and occasional small measures of innovation. Because of such factors, the environment of the Cyberknife closely resembles that of a conventional operating room.

I am convinced that radiosurgery will prove to have a profound impact throughout surgery and radiation oncology, hence my occasional zealotry. Although tumor ablation is the most obvious application for radiosurgery, significant non-neoplastic applications may evolve: for example, radiosurgical trigeminal rhizotomy is already a common procedure, and radiosurgery for temporal lobe epilepsy is being evaluated in a prospective trial. The potential of the CyberKnife to find widespread acceptance within medicine will occur only if the operation of this complex technology can be safely mastered. Again, thorough training is essential if this vision is to be realized.

What Defines Extra-cranial Radiosurgery?

In developing a system for extracranial targeting and treatment, it was critical to begin by defining the specific clinical rationale for such technology. Not surprisingly, it was decided that the specifications for an extracranial radiosurgical system should be consistent with Leksell's original definition for "radiosurgery." In particular, such an instrument should enable the highest possible targeting accuracy (essentially near millimetric RMS errors) and permit ablative doses of radiation to be administered with a maximal use of solid angle for pointing the beam. Very importantly the intent was to administer ablative doses of radiation and thereby enable surgeons to replace open surgical resection or invasive tissue destruction with a non-invasive procedure. This radiosurgical objective is to be distinguished from precision radiation therapy and intensity modulated therapy (IMRT), where accuracy is less important, and conventional fractionation plays a more important role in clinical outcome. An instrument utilizing image-guided robotics seemed uniquely able to achieve these primary surgical objectives.

By extrapolating from the huge prior experience with brain radiosurgery, various surgical specialists are finally in a position to develop new extracranial radiosurgical applications for the CyberKnife. However, similar to other forms of surgery and radiation therapy, the limits of human operative capability are not defined by tools alone. The imagination and diligence with which these instruments are directed towards relieving human suffering are also critical aspects of improving patient outcome.

Cranial Radiosurgery Indications and Patient Selection

Steven D. Chang

Introduction

The CyberKnife, with its frameless robotic image guided system, represents one of the most advanced radiosurgical systems available to date. However, many of the fundamental principals of radiosurgery still apply for determining optimal patient selection and indications for treatment. Several of these principals have been modified during the evolution of the CyberKnife to take full advantage of the system's capabilities. This chapter will discuss criteria used for patient selection for CyberKnife radiosurgery, and will provide an overview of the primary intracranial indications for such treatment.

Patient Selection and Target Criteria
General Patient Characteristics

Generally, there are three characteristics which bear upon patient selection. First, the optimal radiosurgery patient is one with a reasonable estimated survival period after radiosurgery treatment, and most patients with benign tumors easily fall into this category. For patients with malignant disease, survival typically should be on the order of six months or more in order to have significant benefit from treatment. Second, patients should also be able to tolerate treatment, which includes cooperating during setup and actual treatment. We have found that patients with suboptimal attention spans and limited ability to cooperate are difficult to treat, potentially resulting in substantially longer treatment times and possibly larger errors in treatment delivery. Finally, all potential cranial radiosurgery targets should be clearly visible on radiographic treatment planning images. Diffuse, poorly defined targets are not suitable for radiosurgery treatment.

Target Size

As with other radiosurgical systems, lesion size is a factor which determines whether a target is suitable for CyberKnife treatment. In general, 3 cm is thought to be the upper limit of radiosurgical treatment size, although some frame based stereotactic radiosurgery centers have increased the maximum diameter to approximately 3.5 cm. The non-isocentric based nature of the CyberKnife system allows for more homogenous treatments, thereby reducing dosing "hot spots." The maximal dose within the target for a typical Gamma Knife treatment is equal to as much as 200% of the dose to the lesion margin. A typical CyberKnife treatment plan results in a maximal lesion dose of only 125%. The lower maximal dose with respect to lesion margin, along with the option of staging treatment, has allowed us to increase the potential maximal size of the target. While many of our targets are 3 cm or smaller, we have on occasion treated lesions with maximal diameters of 4.5 to 5 cm (with slightly lower dosing than with smaller lesions) with no noticeable increase in complication rates.

Proximity to Critical Structures

Another factor impacting treatment risk is proximity to critical structures. Examples of these structures include the anterior visual pathways, the vestibular and cochlear nerves, and the retina. If the treating physician feels that the target is too close to a particular critical structure, such as the optic chiasm, single fraction frame based treatments may not be an option for some patients. Improved dose homogeneity and the option of staging treatment has allowed the CyberKnife to treat lesions in close proximity to these critical structures, including patients not considered "candidates for radiosurgery" at frame based centers. Our early experience (discussed below) with lesions around the optic apparatus revealed not only that tumor control could be achieved, but that this could be acheived with relatively low risk. Furthermore, several patients had improved vision following treatment.

Staging Treatments

The majority of tumors within the central nervous system can be treated with stereotactic radiosurgery in a single stage. However, some targets, including acoustic neuromas and tumors adjacent to or surrounding the optic apparatus, are adjacent to critical cranial nerves which places these neurologic structures at risk to radiation despite a rapid falloff of dose outside the tumor. The frameless nature of the CyberKnife system allows the option of staged radiosurgery. In this setting, the total dose is delivered in several smaller doses in order to achieve the optimal balance of tumor control and patient safety. Staged treatments allow for the recovery of normal tissues, thereby minimizing normal tissue effects without affecting tumor control rates. Our experience in this regard has focused on staged radiosurgery for the treatment of acoustic neuromas and tumors adjacent to the anterior visual pathways. Both are discussed below.

Indications for Treatment
Acoustic neuromas

Because small to moderate-sized acoustic neuromas typically produce cranial nerve deficits leading to diagnosis, these tumors are ideal targets for radiosurgery. Acoustic neuromas occur as sporadic tumors or as part of the genetic syndrome, type II neurofibromatosis. Although these lesions can be surgically removed, surgery entails a high probability of hearing loss, and a lower, but moderate rate of facial nerve dysfunction. Among 749 patients with acoustic neuroma from three surgical series only 15-37% retained hearing, and approximately 20% had injury to the facial nerve resulting in partial or complete facial palsy (23, 50, 51). Complete resection was achieved in 90% of these cases, and among these tumors, only 1% recurred over five year follow-up. However, 10% recurred over five year follow-up if resection was incomplete (50).

A NIH consensus conference in 1992 recognized the promising role of radiosurgery in the treatment of acoustic neuroma (14). Stereotactic radiosurgery is an effective treatment for small and moderate sized acoustic neuromas, with tumor control rates of 90 to 95% at five to ten year follow-up. Several large series of patients treated with radiosurgery for acoustic neuroma have been compiled (20, 39, 45, 49). Across all of these series, 51% of patients had hearing preserved and more than 90% retained normal facial nerve function (20, 39, 45, 49).

Although the above described results in the radiosurgical treatment of acoustic neuroma represent an improvement in cranial nerve preservation compared to conventional surgery, such patients were treated with single large radiosurgical doses. Recent trends toward delivery of staged radiosurgery and use of lower doses have further increased rates of hearing preservation. In an ongoing series of patients at Stanford treated with three fractions delivered over 36 hours, hearing was preserved in 88% of patients at one year. Hearing maintenance was greater for patients with unilateral tumors than for those with neurofibromatosis type II (100% vs. 71%, p=0.09). Two patients experienced temporary partial facial numbness, but there have been no facial nerve injuries. The radiosurgical endpoint of treatment is reduction or stabilization in tumor size over several years. This result was achieved in 93% of patients reported in the radiosurgical literature (55-63% of tumors decreased and 33-37% stabilized over one year; 78% of tumors decreased over three years) (20, 39, 45, 49). Our experience parallels these results. Patients with recurrent acoustic tumors after resection, and those patients in whom craniotomy is associated with significant risk also represent ideal radiosurgical candidates. Despite the encouraging reports in the literature, follow-up, both in terms of tumor control and complications, is relatively short given the long natural history of acoustic neuroma. Radiosurgery is also limited to treatment of small tumors; large acoustic neuromas must still be treated with surgical resection.

The CyberKnife allows several advances in the treatment of acoustic neuromas. The frameless nature of the system allows more flexibility in the staging of treatment doses. Improved treatment plan software results in improved dose homogeneity and better tumor conformality. Accuracy with this CyberKnife system has been shown to be 1.1 mm, superior to the published accuracy of frame based systems (6).

Pituitary Tumors

Before radiosurgery, treatment of pituitary tumors consisted of surgical resection, medical management with pharmacologic suppression using agents such as bromocriptine and somatostatin, or fractionated external beam radiotherapy. Most pituitary tumors are resectable with a transsphenoidal surgical approach. The recurrence rate after this procedure ranges from 8-15% with mortality rates ranging from 0.3 to 1.8% (13, 37, 46, 52). Among hormone secreting pituitary tumors, hormonal control rates range from 42-86% depending upon the type of hormone secreted (13, 37, 46, 52). Morbidity and mortality rates following surgical resection of pituitary tumors are higher among patients with recurrent disease or with significant intercurrent medical conditions. Radiosurgery is a particularly attractive alternative to resection in these settings.

There is considerable experience with the use of fractionated radiotherapy for managing pituitary tumors. When this treatment is used alone, ten year tumor control rates for pituitary tumors range from 77 to 87% (26, 70). However, the rates of hypopituitarism in one study were 35% for thyroxine, 32% for glucocorticoids, and 33% for sex hormones (70). While 56% of these patients required additional medical management, biochemical hormonal control in this group was 39% at 10 years (71). Overall complication rates from fractionated radiotherapy range from 3 to 7%, and generally involve injuries to the visual tracts, late secondary malignancies, and rare vascular injuries (18, 70).

Although several small series report high control rates after radiosurgery for small primary or recurrent pituitary tumors (22, 64, 65, 72), follow-up has been limited to two to five years. Reported rates of recurrence range from 0-2%. Hormonal cure rates after radiosurgery have been reported to range from 48-100% depending on the subtype of tumor (22, 64, 65, 72). Treatment is most successful for patients with prolactinoma, acromegaly, and Cushing's disease, and treatment is least effective in rare cases of Nelson's syndrome.

Large pituitary tumors (greater than 3.5 cm), or those tumors closer than 3 mm to the optic nerve or chiasm cannot be treated by single staged radiosurgery without a significant risk of radiation injury to the optic apparatus. Alternative strategies for such patients include 1) combined surgical resection and radiosurgery (with radiosurgery reserved for treatment of any residual sellar and cavernous sinus tumor once it has been debulked away from the optic apparatus), 2) conventional external beam irradiation, or 3) staged CyberKnife radiosurgery. Regardless of treatment, all patients require serial endocrinologic studies to document changes in hormonal function, so that hormonal replacement can be instituted if hypopituitarism develops. Patients with recurrent pituitary adenoma after fractionated radiotherapy to the pituitary region may be treatable with radiosurgery, although the risks for radiation injury are not well defined in this setting.

Malignant Glioma Boosts

The outcome with current therapy for malignant gliomas is, by virtually any standard, poor. Nevertheless, primary treatment of this tumor consists of surgical resection, when possible, followed by fractionated external beam radiotherapy. Such therapy results in a mean survival on the order of 9 months (59). Adjuvant chemotherapy has been used with mixed results. Small tumors have been approached with radiation dose escalation using either brachytherapy or radiosurgery with some encouraging results (28, 78).

Recent studies have evaluated the effectiveness of stereotactic radiosurgical boost to areas of contrast enhancement, in conjunction with fractionated radiotherapy, for the treatment of malignant gliomas (4, 31, 36). Patient selection criteria include a high performance level and tumor diameter less than 3.5 cm. In a recent Gamma Knife series of 189 glioma patients who received a median tumor boost dose of 16 Gy (range 8-30 Gy) delivered to a median volume of 5.9 cc (range 1.3-52 cc), the median survival was 86 weeks if the tumor was small and unifocal. In contrast, the median survival was reported to be 40 weeks for larger and more diffuse tumors (36). A second Gamma Knife series of 64 glioblastoma multiforme and 43 anaplastic astrocytoma patients (all with tumors less than 3.5 cm maximal diameter) treated with a mean of 15.5 Gy to the tumor margin (mean of 15.2 Gy for anaplastic astrocytomas) revealed an improved survival benefit when compared to historical control (31). In this series of patients with malignant gliomas, median survival following diagnosis and radiosurgery was 26 and 16 months respectively for glioblastoma multiforme and 32 and 21 months respectively for anaplastic astrocytoma (31). A LINAC series of 11 patients with high grade glioma used a dose of 12.5 Gy delivered to a median treatment volume of 14 cm^3. Although all patients had progression of intracranial disease within one year of radiosurgery, an actuarial survival of 17 months was reported (4). From these studies, it appears that radiosurgical boost doses for malignant gliomas result in a modest increase in patient survival. Nevertheless, this increased survival may relate to pre-radiosurgical Karnofsky status, patient age, and tumor volume (4, 31, 36).

Often residual or recurrent high grade gliomas have irregular shapes and volumes. The ability to use non-isocentric treatment planning to conform to such irregular shapes is one of the primary advantages of the CyberKnife. Staged radiosurgery has proved useful in treating lower grade gliomas around the optic chiasm, with results comparable to conventional radiotherapy.

Metastatic Tumors

The treatment of brain metastases is the most common application of radiosurgery due to the high incidence of this disease. The American Cancer Society estimates that 170,000 cancer patients develop cerebral metastases each year in the United States (55). Because most patients with metastases eventually succumb to their underlying malignancy, the primary benefits of radiosurgery are palliation of symptoms and some modest prolongation of survival. Median survival after radiosurgery (6.4-10 months) (9, 15, 19, 30, 40, 60, 64, 66, 73) is comparable to surgical resection followed by conventional fractionated radiotherapy (4-13 months) (17, 67), with good local control (9, 15, 19, 30, 40, 60, 64, 66, 73). Two studies have shown that patients treated with radiosurgery for either one or two brain metastases have equivalent, prolonged survival similar to that achieved with surgical resection (1, 29).

Selection criteria for radiosurgery generally include: 1) a limited number of brain metastases (typically less than or equal to 3, 2) maximal tumor diameter less than 3.5 cm for each lesion, 3) suitable target shape, 4) absent or stable disease at the primary and other extracranial sites. There are two clinical situations in which surgical resection may be preferable to radiosurgery for treatment of brain metastases; when the primary source is unknown, and when there are significant symptoms attributable to mass effect and edema unrelieved by corticosteroids. Surgical resection typically relieves symptoms more promptly than radiosurgery.

Radiosurgery is preferable to surgery for patients whose medical condition precludes craniotomy, for patients with tumors located in eloquent cerebral regions, and for patients who refuse surgery. Radiosurgery avoids the morbidity and mortality in the perioperative period that craniotomy entails. Furthermore, several tumors can be radiated during one outpatient treatment. Radiosurgical ablation of brain metastases can be followed by whole brain fractionated radiotherapy to minimize the likelihood of regional recurrence. However, radiosurgery can also be used without subsequent whole brain radiotherapy in patients with one to three metastases. Unlike conventional brain irradiation, radiosurgery can be repeated for metachronous lesions months to years after initial treatment. Because most brain metastases are treated with a single dose of radiosurgery, indications for treatment and results with the CyberKnife are comparable to other radiosurgical systems. Exceptions include metastases within the anterior visual pathways, which can be treated with staged radiosurgery, and broad dural based metastases which can be easily treated using the non-isocentric based software of the CyberKnife system.

Boost for Nasopharyngeal Carcinoma

Nasopharyngeal carcinoma (NPC) arises in the mucosa or submucosa of the nasopharynx, and frequently spreads to the skull base. Given the radiosensitivity of the tumor, radiotherapy (XRT) is the primary treatment. However, there is a significant incidence of local failure (26-100%) in more advanced NPC after treatment with conventional XRT (57, 75, 76). Higher XRT doses or brachytherapy boosts increase local control (38, 56, 75-77) but the possibility of normal tissue injury increases. Furthermore, the inability to effectively treat tumor extension to the skull base is a limitation of these techniques. Because of the historically high local failure rate, we developed a protocol to deliver a planned stereotactic radiosurgical boost following conventional radiation therapy in patients with nasopharyngeal carcinoma.

All patients with biopsy-proven NPC received standard XRT to a total dose to the nasopharynx of 66 Gy, utilizing 200 cGy daily treatments. Elective neck irradiation to a dose of 50 Gy was also used; involved lymph nodes received XRT boosts to a total dose of 66 Gy. Most patients received cisplatinum-based chemotherapy as an additional part of their treatment. Patients were then treated with radiosurgery within four weeks of completing XRT. The prescribed dose of radiation was administered to the periphery of the original lesion, corresponding to the 80-85% isodose contour. The median dose was 12 Gy (range of 7 to 15 Gy). Mean follow-up approximates 30 months for the 45 patients receiving this treatment. Throughout the course of follow-up, no local recurrences occurred among the 45 patients with NPC treated with radiosurgery. Two patients developed late complications following radiosurgery consisting of radiation edema in the adjacent mesial temporal lobe.

Our preliminary experience shows that a high rate of local control can be achieved even in advanced staged NPC patients with stereotactic radiosurgery. We believe that radiosurgery is more effective in such cases than brachytherapy because of the ability of radiosurgery to effectively treat the base of skull. While intracavitary brachytherapy in the nasopharynx is likely to be effective in treating tumors confined to the mucosa or submucosa, it is unlikely to eradicate a larger mass that extends several centimeters beneath the mucosal surface. Radiosurgery provides not only the same benefits as brachytherapy (i.e., relative sparing of normal tissues and the ability to safely boost regions of involvement to high doses) but it is also able to deliver a high radiation dose to those sites remote from the nasopharynx. Based on this experience, patients with advanced NPC treated at Stanford receive a 66 Gy XRT dose with concurrent cisplatinum chemotherapy, followed by a 12 Gy radiosurgery to the primary site, after which three more cycles of cisplatinum/5-FU chemotherapy are given.

Arteriovenous Malformations

Arteriovenous malformations (AVMs) are abnormal clusters of blood vessels that directly shunt blood between arteries and veins without the normal intervening capillary system. Patients with these lesions present with symptoms such as hemorrhage, seizures, headaches, or progressive neurologic deficits. The annual rate of hemorrhage for angiographically visible AVMs is estimated to be 3-4% per year, while the risk of death is 1% per year (3). For decades, surgical resection has been the primary treatment for AVMs. Recent advances in microsurgical techniques have substantially decreased morbidity and mortality; large published series indicate a 90-99% rate of cure, with an associated 8-18% risk of serious morbidity and 1-5% risk of mortality (25, 48, 53, 61, 80). Despite the success of surgical resection, stereotactic radiosurgery is an important alternative for small to moderately sized AVMs, particularly those located in surgically inaccessible regions or in patients who are poor operative candidates (3, 41, 62, 63). The primary mechanism of AVM obliteration following radiosurgery involves hyperplasia of the vascular intima (7), with progressive narrowing and, ultimately, occlusion. Such obliteration typically takes place over two to three years. AVMs of less than 4 cm in diameter treated with 20-25 Gy have a 3 year obliteration rate of 76-95% with relatively modest morbidity (2.5-4.5% permanent neurologic deficits, 2.5-4.5% transient deficits) (3, 10, 21, 34, 41, 62, 63, 68).

There are three considerations when weighing surgery versus radiosurgery for treatment of AVMs. First, AVMs greater than 4 cm diameter have only a 33-50% rate of obliteration at three years after radiosurgery but a 20-30% complication rate following treatment doses of 15-20 Gy (3, 62, 63). The rate of obliteration is increased for larger AVMs by using higher doses (25-45 Gy); however, the risk of radiation-induced complications increases significantly. Another important disadvantage of radiosurgery is that the risk of intracranial hemorrhage persists during the interval between treatment and complete obliteration (3, 41, 62, 63). Also, serial radiographic studies including cerebral angiograms are necessary to confirm complete obliteration. Despite these limitations, radiosurgery appears to have less morbidity than surgical resection in those patients with high risk AVMs in eloquent brain.

The CyberKnife system allows treatment of these same AVMs in a frameless fashion. Treatment planning is performed on CT imaging or on CT/MR fusions in a volumetric fashion. Doses utilized are similar to frame based systems. The advent of 3-dimensional rotational angiography represents a breakthrough for CyberKnife radiosurgery of AVMs. Such digital rotational images can be utilized on the CyberKnife to treat AVMs, thus overcoming many of the targeting errors of treating AVMs with 2-dimensional angiographic films.

Trigeminal Neuralgia

Trigeminal neuralgia is a disease which has been successfully treated with the CyberKnife. There exists substantial literature on radiosurgery for trigeminal neuralgia (24, 35, 42, 54, 58). Several issues arise when using the CyberKnife to target an object as small as the trigeminal nerve. First, accuracy of the system is critical, as a 1.5 mm error when treating a 3 mm target could result in a 50% total error in dose delivery. While it is frameless, the CyberKnife has accuracy comparable to existing frame based systems (6). Furthermore, in order to avoid the potential increase in error as a result of MR/CT fusions, we typically treat patients using only a CT scan obtained after intrathecal injection of metrizamide. This creates a CT image similar to appearance of a T2 MRI sequence without the fusion error introduced with a fusion algorithm.

Second, the non-isocentric nature of the CyberKnife treatment planning software allows a more ovoid target distribution to be delivered to the nerve.

While others have utilized multiple isocenters to extend the length of the nerve treated with radiosurgery, they have not shown that this improves resolution of symptoms. In our experience, we have achieved rapid resolution of pain, often on the order of 24 hours, with no substantial difference in side effects compared to frame based series.

Our protocol for trigeminal neuralgia treatment planning is to treat an approximately 6 to 8 mm segment of the trigeminal nerve 3 mm beyond the emergence of the nerve from the brainstem. Our dose to the periphery of our defined nerve target is 60 to 66 Gy, with a maximal dose within the target of 68 to 76 Gy. Note that, while our radiosurgery dose to the nerve periphery is lower than most frame based series, in our experience, the longer segment of nerve treated offsets this lower dose and produces pain relief within 24 hours.

References

1. Alexander E, Moriarty TM, Davis RB, Wen PY, Fine HA, Black PM, Kooy HM, Loeffler JS: Stereotactic radiosurgery for the definitive, noninvasive treatment of brain metastasis. J Nat Cancer Inst 87:34-40, 1995.
2. Barbaro NM, Gutin PH, Wilson CB, Sheline GE, Boldrey EB, Wara WM: Radiation therapy in the treatment of partially resected meningiomas. Neurosurgery 20:525-528, 1987.
3. Brown RD, Jr., Wiebers DO, Forbes G, O'Fallon WM, Piepgras DG, Marsh WR, Maciunas RJ: The natural history of unruptured intracranial arteriovenous malformations. J Neurosurg 68:352-357, 1988.
4. Buatti JM, Friedman WA, Bova FJ, Mendenhall WM: Linac radiosurgery for high-grade gliomas: The University of Florida experience. Int J Radiat Oncol Biol Phys 32:205-210, 1995.
5. Chang SD, Adler JR: Treatment of cranial base meningiomas with linear accelerator radiosurgery. Neurosurgery 41:1019-1027, 1997.
6. Chang SD, Main W, Martin DP, Gibbs IC, Heilbrun MP: An analysis of the accuracy of the CyberKnife: A robotic frameless stereotactic radiosurgical system. Neurosurgery 52:140-147, 2003.
7. Chang SD, Shuster DL, Steinberg GK, Levy RP, Frankel KA: Stereotactic radiosurgery of arteriovenous malformations: Pathologic changes in resected tissue. Clinical Neuropathology 16:111-116, 1997.
8. Ciric I, Landau B: Tentorial and posterior cranial fossa meningiomas: operative results and long term follow up: experience with 26 cases. Surg Neurology 39:530-537, 1993.
9. Coffey RJ, Flickinger JC, Bissonette DJ, Lunsford LD: Radiosurgery for solitary brain metastases using the cobalt-60 gamma unit: methods and results in 24 patients. Int J Radiat Oncol Biol Phys 20:1287-1295, 1991.
10. Colombo F, Pozza F, Chierego G, Casentini L, De Luca G, Francescon P: Linear accelerator radiosurgery of cerebral arteriovenous malformations: An update. Neurosurgery 34:14-21, 1994.
11. DeMonte F, Smith HK, al-Mefty O: Outcome of aggressive removal of cavernous sinus meningiomas. J Neurosurg 81:245-251, 1994.
12. Duma CM, Lunsford LD, Kondziolka D, Harsh GRt, Flickinger JC: Stereotactic radiosurgery of cavernous sinus meningiomas as an addition or alternative to microsurgery. Neurosurgery 32:699-704; discussion 704-695, 1993.
13. Dyer EH, Civit T, Visot A, Delalande O, Derome P: Transsphenoidal surgery for pituitary adenomas in children. Neurosurgery 34:207-212; discussion 212, 1994.
14. Eldridge R, Parry D: Vestibular schwannoma (acoustic neuroma). Consensus development conference [see comments]. Neurosurgery 30:962-964, 1992.
15. Engenhart R, Kimmig BN, Hover KH, Wowra B, Romahn J, Lorenz WJ, van Kaick G, Wannenmacher M: Long-term follow-up for brain metastases treated by percutaneous stereotactic single high-dose irradiation. Cancer 71:1353-1361, 1993.
16. Engenhart R, Kimmig BN, Hover KH, Wowra B, Sturm V, van Kaick G, Wannenmacher M: Stereotactic single high dose radiation therapy of benign intracranial meningiomas. Int J Radiat Oncol Biol Phys 19:1021-1026, 1990.
17. Ferrara M, Bizzozzero L, Talamonti G, D'Angelo VA: Surgical treatment of 100 single brain metastases. Analysis of the results. J Neurosurg Sci 34:303-308, 1990.
18. Fisher BJ, Gaspar LE, Noone B: Radiation therapy of pituitary adenoma: Delayed sequelae. Radiology 187:843-846, 1993.
19. Flickinger JC, Kondziolka D, Lunsford LD, Coffey RJ, Goodman ML, Shaw EG, Hudgins WR, Weiner R, Harsh GR, Sneed PK: A multi-institutional experience with stereotactic radiosurgery for solitary brain metastasis [see comments]. Int J Radiat Oncol Biol Phys 28:797-802, 1994.
20. Flickinger JC, Lunsford LD, Linskey ME, Duma CM, Kondziolka D: Gamma knife radiosurgery for acoustic tumors: multivariate analysis of four year results. Radiother Oncol 27:91-98, 1993.
21. Friedman WA, Bova FJ, Mendenhall WM: Linear accelerator radiosurgery for arteriovenous malformations: The relationship of size to outcome. J Neurosurg 82:180-189, 1995.
22. Ganz JC, Backlund EO, Thorsen FA: The effects of Gamma Knife surgery of pituitary adenomas on tumor growth and endocrinopathies. Stereotact Funct Neurosurg 61 Suppl 1:30-37, 1993.
23. Glasscock ME, Hays JW, Minor LB, Haynes DS, Carrasco VN: Preservation of hearing in surgery for acoustic neuromas [see comments]. J Neurosurg 78:864-870, 1993.
24. Hasegawa T, Kondziolka D, Spior R, Flickinger JC, Lunsford LD: Repeat radiosurgery for refractory trigeminal neuralgia. Neurosurgery 50:494-502, 2002.
25. Heros RC, Korosue K, Diebold PM: Surgical excision of cerebral arteriovenous malformations: late results. Neurosurgery 26:570-577; discussion 577-578, 1990.
26. Hughes MN, Lamas KJ, Yelland ME, Tripcony LB: Pituitary adenomas: Long-term results for radiotherapy alone and postoperative radiotherapy. Int J Rad Onc Biol Phys 27:1035-1043, 1993.
27. Jaaskelainen J: Seemingly complete removal of histologically benign intracranial meningioma: late recurrence rate and factors predicting recurrence in 657 patients. A multivariate analysis. Surg Neurol 26:461-469, 1986.
28. Jeremic B, Grujicic D, Antunovic V, Djuric L, Shibamoto Y: Accelerated hyperfractionated radiation therapy for malignant glioma. A phase II study. Amer J Clin Oncol 18:449-453, 1995.
29. Joseph J, Adler JR, Cox RS, Hancock SL: Linear accelerator-based stereotactic radiosurgery for brain metastases: The influence of number of lesions on survival. J Clin Oncol 14:1085-1092, 1996.
30. Kihlstrom L, Karlsson B, Lindquist C: Gamma Knife surgery for cerebral metastases. Implications for survival based on 16 years experience. Stereotact Funct Neurosurg 61 Suppl 1:45-50, 1993.

31. Kondziolka D, Flickinger JC, Bissonette DJ, Bozik M, Lunsford LD: Survival benefit of stereotactic radiosurgery for patients with malignant glial neoplasms. Neurosurgery 41:776-785, 1997.
32. Kondziolka D, Lunsford LD: Radiosurgery of meningiomas. Neurosurg Clin N Am 3:219-230, 1992.
33. Kondziolka D, Lunsford LD, Coffey RJ, Flickinger JC: Stereotactic radiosurgery of meningiomas. J Neurosurg 74:552-559, 1991.
34. Kondziolka D, Lunsford LD, Flickinger J: Gamma knife stereotactic radiosurgery for cerebral vascular malformations, in Alexander E, Loeffler JS, Lunsford LD (eds): *Stereotactic Radiosurgery.* New York, McGraw-Hill, 1993, pp 136-146.
35. Kondziolka D, Lunsford LD, Flickinger JC: Stereotactic radiosurgery for the treatment of trigeminal neuralgia. Clin J Pain 18:42-47, 2002.
36. Larson DA, Gutin PH, McDermott M, Lamborn K, Sneed PK, Wara WM, Flickinger JC, Kondziolka D, Lunsford LD, Hudgins WR: Gamma knife for glioma: Selection factors and survival. Int J Rad Onc Biol Phys 36:1045-1053, 1996.
37. Laws E: Surgical management of pituitary tumors, in E. M, Samaan N (eds): *Endocrine Tumors.* Boston, Blackwell Scientific Publishers, 1993, pp 215-222.
38. Levendag PC, Schmitz PI, Jansen PP, Senan S, Eijkenboom WM, Sipkema D, Meeuwis CA, Kolkman-Deurloo IK, Visser AG: Fractionated high-dose-rate and pulsed-dose-rate brachytherapy: first clinical experience in squamous cell carcinoma of the tonsillar fossa and soft palate. Int J Radiat Oncol Biol Phys 38:497-506, 1997.
39. Lindquist C, Steiner L: Radiosurgery for tumors, in Wilkins R, Rengachary S (eds): *Neurosurgery.* New York, McGraw-Hill, 1995, p 185.
40. Loeffler J, Alexander III E: Radiosurgery for the treatment of intracranial metastasis, in Alexander III E, Loeffler J, Lunsford LD (eds): *Stereotactic Radiosurgery.* New York, McGraw-Hill, 1993, pp 197-206.
41. Lunsford LD, Kondziolka D, Bissonette DJ, Maitz AH, Flickinger JC: Stereotactic radiosurgery of brain vascular malformations. Neurosurg Clin N Am 3:79-98, 1992.
42. Lunsford LD, Young RF: Radiosurgery for trigeminal neuralgia. Surg Neurol 54:285-287, 2000.
43. Mahmood A, Qureshi NH, Malik GM: Intracranial meningiomas: analysis of recurrence after surgical treatment. Acta Neurochiurgica 126:53-58, 1994.
44. Mehta MP, Rozental JM, Levin AB, Mackie TR, Kubsad SS, Gehring MA, Kinsella TJ: Defining the role of radiosurgery in the management of brain metastases. Int J Radiat Oncol Biol Phys 24:619-625, 1992.
45. Mendenhall WM, Friedman WA, Bova FJ: Linear accelerator-based stereotactic radiosurgery for acoustic schwannomas [see comments]. Int J Radiat Oncol Biol Phys 28:803-810, 1994.
46. Mindermann T, Wilson CB: Pediatric pituitary adenomas. Neurosurgery 36:259-268; discussion 269, 1995.
47. Miralbell R, Linggood RM, de la Monte S, Convery K, Munzenrider JE, Mirimanoff RO: The role of radiotherapy in the treatment of subtotally resected benign meningiomas. J Neurooncol 13:157-164, 1992.
48. Morgan MK, Johnston IH, Hallinan JM, Weber NC: Complications of surgery for arteriovenous malformations of the brain [see comments]. J Neurosurg 78:176-182, 1993.
49. Noren G, Greitz D, Hirsch A, Lax I: Gamma knife surgery in acoustic tumours. Acta Neurochir Suppl (Wien) 58:104-107, 1993.
50. Ojemann RG: Management of acoustic neuromas (vestibular schwannomas) (honored guest presentation). Clin Neurosurg 40:498-535, 1993.
51. Pellet W, Emram B, Cannoni M, Pech A, Zanaret M, Thomassin M: [Functional results of the surgery of unilateral acoustic neuroma]. Neurochirurgie 39:24-40; discussion 40-21, 1993.
52. Petruson B, Jakobsson KE, Elfverson J, Bengtsson BA: Five-year follow-up of nonsecreting pituitary adenomas. Arch Otolaryngol Head Neck Surg 121:317-322, 1995.
53. Piepgras DG, Sundt TM, Jr., Ragoowansi AT, Stevens L: Seizure outcome in patients with surgically treated cerebral arteriovenous malformations. J Neurosurg 78:5-11, 1993.
54. Pollock BE, Phuong LK, Gorman DA, Foote RL, Stafford SL: Stereotactic radiosurgery for idiopathic trigeminal neuralgia. J Neurosurg 97:347-353, 2002.
55. Posner J: Management of brain metastases. Rev Neurol 148:477-487, 1992.
56. Qin DX, Hu YH, Yan JH, Xu GZ, Cai WM, Wu XL, Cao DX, Gu XZ: Analysis of 1379 patients with nasopharyngeal carcinoma treated by radiation. Cancer 61:1117-1124, 1988.
57. Sanguineti G, Geara FB, Garden AS, Tucker SL, Ang KK, Morrison WH, Peters LJ: Carcinoma of the nasopharynx treated by radiotherapy alone: determinants of local and regional control. Int J Radiat Oncol Biol Phys 37:985-996, 1997.
58. Shetter AG, Rogers CL, Ponce F, Fiedler JA, Smith K, Speiser BL: Gamma knife radiosurgery for recurrent trigeminal neuralgia. J Neurosurg 97:536-538, 2002.
59. Simpson JR, Horton J, Scott C, Curran WJ, Rubin P, Fischbach J, Isaacson S, Rotman M, Asbell SO, Nelson JS: Influence of location and extent of surgical resection on survival of patients with glioblastoma multiforme: results of three consecutive Radiation Therapy Oncology Group (RTOG) clinical trials. Int J Radiat Oncol Biol Phys 26:239-244, 1993.
60. Somaza S, Kondziolka D, Lunsford LD, Kirkwood JM, Flickinger JC: Stereotactic radiosurgery for cerebral metastatic melanoma. J Neurosurg 79:661-666, 1993.
61. Stein BM: Arteriovenous malformations of the medial cerebral hemisphere and the limbic system. J Neurosurg 60:23-31, 1984.
62. Steinberg GK, Fabrikant JI, Marks MP, Levy RP, Frankel KA, Phillips MH, Shuer LM, Silverberg GD: Stereotactic heavy-charged-particle Bragg-peak radiation for intracranial arteriovenous malformations [see comments]. N Engl J Med 323:96-101, 1990.
63. Steiner L, Lindquist C, Adler JR, Torner JC, Alves W, Steiner M: Clinical outcome of radiosurgery for cerebral arteriovenous malformations. J Neurosurg 77:1-8, 1992.
64. Steiner L, Prasad D, Lindquist C, Karlsson B, Steiner M: Gamma knife surgery in vascular, neoplastic, and functional disorders of the nervous system, in Schmidek HH, Sweet WH (eds): *Operative Neurosurgical Techniques.* Philadelphia, W. B. Saunders, 1994, pp 667-694.
65. Stephanian E, Lunsford LD, Coffey RJ, Bissonette DJ, Flickinger JC: Gamma knife surgery for sellar and suprasellar tumors. Neurosurg Clin N Am 3:207-218, 1992.
66. Sturm V, Kimmig B, Engenhardt R, Schlegel W, Pastyr O, Treuer H, Schabbert S, Voges J: Radiosurgical treatment of cerebral metastases. Method, indications and results. Stereotact Funct Neurosurg 57:7-10, 1991.
67. Sundaresan N, Galicich JH: Surgical treatment of brain metastases. Clinical and computerized tomography evaluation of the results of treatment. Cancer 55:1382-1388, 1985.
68. Sutcliffe JC, Forster DM, Walton L, Dias PS, Kemeny AA: Untoward clinical effects after stereotactic radiosurgery for intracranial arteriovenous malformations. Br J Neurosurg 6:177-185, 1992.
69. Thoren M: Stereotactic radiosurgery with the cobalt-60 gamma unit in the treatment of growth hormone-producing pituitary tumors. Neurosurgery 29:663-668, 1991.
70. Tsang RW, Brierley JD, Panzarella T, Gospodarowicz MK, Sutcliffe SB, Simpson WJ: Radiation therapy for pituitary adenoma: Treatment outcome and prognostic factors. Int J Rad Onc Biol Phys 30:557-565, 1994.
71. Tsang RW, Brierley JD, Panzarella T, Gospodarowicz MK, Sutcliffe SB, Simpson WJ: Role of radiation therapy in clinical

hormonally active pituitary adenomas. Radiotherapy and Oncol 41:45-53, 1996.

72. Valentino V: Postoperative radiosurgery of pituitary adenomas. J Neurosurg Sci 35:207-211, 1991.

73. Valentino V, Mirri MA, Schinaia G, Dalle Ore G: Linear accelerator and Greitz-Bergstrom's head fixation system in radiosurgery of single cerebral metastases. A report of 86 cases. Acta Neurochir (Wien) 121:140-145, 1993.

74. Valentino V, Schinaia G, Raimondi AJ: The results of radiosurgical management of 72 middle fossa meningiomas. Acta Neurochir (Wien) 122:60-70, 1993.

75. Vikram B, Mishra UB, Strong EW, Manolatos S: Patterns of failure in carcinoma of the nasopharynx: I. Failure at the primary site. Int J Radiat Oncol Biol Phys 11:1455-1459, 1985.

76. Wang CC: Improved local control of nasopharyngeal carcinoma after intracavitary brachytherapy boost. Am J Clin Oncol 14:5-8, 1991.

CyberKnife Radiosurgery for the Spine

Peter C. Gerszten
William C. Welch

Radiotherapy for Spinal Lesions

Standard treatment options for spinal tumors include radiotherapy alone, radionuclide therapy, radiotherapy plus systemic chemotherapy, hormonal therapy, or surgical decompression and/or stabilization followed by radiotherapy (1). If a spinal tumor causes compression of the spinal cord or other neural elements, surgical decompression is often necessary with or without spinal fixation based on the extent of spinal column destruction and instability of the spine. The goals of local radiation therapy in the treatment of spinal tumors have been palliation of pain, prevention of pathologic fractures, and halting progression of, or reversing neurological compromise.

The role of radiation therapy in the treatment of tumors of the spine has been well established. A primary factor that limits radiation dose in tumor control with conventional radiotherapy is the low tolerance of the spinal cord to radiation. However, conventional external beam radiotherapy lacks the precision to allow delivery of large doses of radiation near radiosensitive structures such as the spinal cord. It is the low tolerance of the spinal cord to radiation that often limits the treatment dose to a level that is far below the optimal therapeutic dose (2, 3, 4).

If the radiation dose could be confined more precisely to the treatment volume, as is the case for intracranial radiosurgery, the likelihood of successful tumor control should increase at the same time that the risk of spinal cord injury decreases. Recent studies using hypofractionated or single dose treatments for spinal metastases reported results that were comparable to conventional fractionation (5, 6). Furthermore, hypofractionation or single dose radiation decreases the treatment duration, is more convenient for patients, and is less costly.

Spinal Radiosurgery

Current frame-based stereotactic radiosurgery devices do not have the capability of treating lesions below the foramen magnum using skull fixation devices. Conformal radiotherapy and intensity-modulated radiation therapy (IMRT) are limited by problems with target immobilization. This limitation of IMRT precludes large single fraction treatment to spinal lesions. Treatment of spinal lesions by stereotactic conformal radiotherapy and IMRT have shown promising clinical results (7). Conventional frame-based devices used for stereotactic radiosurgery for intracranial lesions use a rigid frame to immobilize the lesion at a known location in space. The frame acts as a fiducial reference system to provide accurate targeting and delivery of the radiation dose. Intracranial radiosurgery is practical because the lesions are fixed with respect to the cranium, which can be immobilized rigidly in a stereotactic frame. Spinal lesions also have a fixed relationship to the spine. However, stereotactic radiosurgery techniques developed for spinal lesions using standard linear accelerators require the placement of an invasive rigid external frame system directly to the spine (8). In order to improve reproducibility in stereotactic irradiation without using an immobilization device or body frame, the prototype of an integrated computed tomography-linac irradiation system connecting a CT scanner and linac via a common treatment couch has been developed (9). This device, however, has not been tested clinically.

The use of multiple beams of radiation requires extremely precise control of position and movement of the linear accelerator. Traditional stereotactic radiosurgery is limited to intracranial disease because precise localization can be achieved only by neurosurgical frames fixed to the patient's skull. Most radiosurgery techniques involve the fixation of a head frame device that is attached by four screws to the patient's skull. This device insures precise targeting of the radiation to the tumor. As a corollary, treatment is typically limited to single fraction treatments. Radiosurgery has been reported in the treatment of many different intracranial pathologies, both benign and malignant, and is widely accepted as safe and effective (6, 10, 11, 12, 13, 14).

Stereotactic radiosurgery offers a method for delivering a high dose of radiation in a single or limited number of fractions to a small volume encompassing the tumor while minimizing the dose to adjacent normal structures. A study from the University of Arizona in 1996 demonstrated that stereotactic radiosurgery to the spine using a body frame was both feasible and safe (8). However, precise targeting of the tumor required that the spine be fixed using a large frame with clamps applied to the spinous processes. Multiple one to two centimeter incisions under general anesthesia were necessary. Although the study concluded that radiosurgery was beneficial, the overall treatment strategy was associated with risks from spinous process fractures, infection, delayed wound healing, and anesthesia.

A new image-guided frameless stereotactic radiosurgery delivery system known as the CyberKnife® (Accuray, Inc., Sunnyvale, CA) has been developed that was approved by the United States Food and Drug Administration in 2001 for use throughout the entire spine. The CyberKnife was first developed for treatment of brain tumors at Stanford University. Since 1994, the device has been used at a number of sites around the world to treat a variety of benign and malignant intracranial lesions (15, 16). As expected, treatment outcome has closely mirrored the results of conventional frame-based radiosurgery (3). With the ability to treat lesions outside of the skull using fiducial tracking, a growing interest in the treatment of spinal lesions using the CyberKnife has emerged (3, 17, 18).

The CyberKnife System

The CyberKnife (Accuray, Inc., Sunnyvale, CA) system consists of a lightweight linear accelerator mounted on a robotic arm.

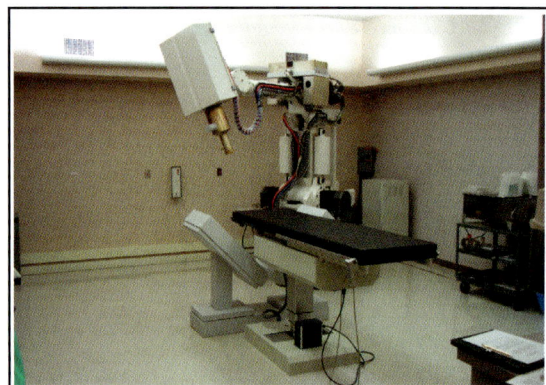

Figure 1. The CyberKnife Radiosurgery System. Note the two amorphous silicon x-ray screens positioned orthogonally to the treatment couch. The couch can move to position the fiducials in front of the cameras.

Real-time imaging tracking allows for patient movement tracking with 1 mm spatial accuracy (3, 19, 20). The CyberKnife was developed as a non-invasive means to precisely align treatment beams with targets. It differs from conventional frame-based radiosurgery in three fundamental ways (3). First, it references the position of the treatment target to internal radiographic features such as the skull or implanted fiducials rather than a frame. Second, it uses real-time x-ray imaging to establish the position of the lesion during treatment and then dynamically brings the radiation beam into alignment with the observed position of the treatment target. Third, it aims each beam independently, without a fixed isocenter. Changes in patient position during the treatment are compensated for by adaptive beam pointing rather than controlled through rigid immobilization. This allows the patient to be positioned comfortably in the treatment room without precise reproduction of the position in the treatment planning study. Because of the spatial precision with which the CyberKnife can administer radiation, it is theoretically feasible to administer a tumoricidal radiation dose in a single outpatient treatment. By minimizing the irradiation of surrounding healthy tissue, it should also be possible to decrease the rate of complications.

The CyberKnife consists of a computer controlled, compact source of high energy x-rays, that is smaller and lighter in weight than linear accelerators used in conventional radiotherapy (21, 22, 23, 24). The smaller size allows it to be mounted on a computer-controlled six-axis robotic manipulator that permits a much wider range of beam orientations than can be achieved with conventional radiotherapy devices.

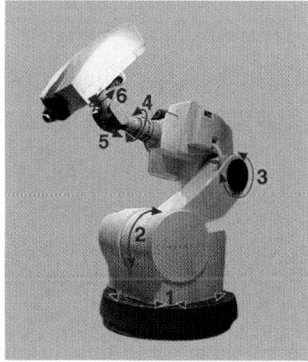

Figure 2. The CyberKnife consists of a linear accelerator mounted on a six-axis robotic manipulator that permits a wide range of beam orientations.

The CyberKnife system utilizes image-guided frameless robotic radiosurgery. Two ceiling mounted diagnostic x-ray cameras are positioned orthogonally (90-degree offset) to acquire real-time images of the patient's internal anatomy during treatment. The images are gathered using two amorphous silicon x-ray screens capable of generating high-resolution digital images (25). The images are processed automatically to identify radiographic features, then registered to the treatment planning study to measure the position of the treatment site. The measured position is communicated through a real-time control loop to a robotic manipulator that aims a compact 6 MV linear accelerator.

The system can adapt to changes in patient position during treatment by acquiring targeting images repeatedly and then adjusting the direction of the treatment beam. The target to be treated is identified prior to treatment on planning images. Between 150 and 200 beams are used to irradiate the target in a stereotactic fashion. The treatment beam can be maneuvered and pointed nearly anywhere in space. Treatment beams also are not confined to isocentric geometry, so they can be arranged in complex overlapping patterns that conform to irregularly shaped tumor volumes (3). An analysis of the accuracy of the CyberKnife radiosurgery system found that the machine has a clinically relevant accuracy of 1.1 ± 0.3 mm using a 1.25mm CT slice thickness. Hence, the CyberKnife precision is comparable to published localization errors in other current frame-based radiosurgical systems (25).

Indications for Spine Radiosurgery

The indications for spine radiosurgery using the CyberKnife are currently evolving and will continue to evolve as clinical experience increases. This is similar to the evolution of indications for intracranial radiosurgery that occurred during the 1990s. Table 1 summarizes the candidate lesions for CyberKnife spine radiosurgery. Similar to cranial radiosurgery, candidate lesions may be of either benign or malignant histology. Spinal vascular malformations are also amenable to spinal radiosurgery (3).

> **Table 1**
> **Candidate lesions for CyberKnife radiosurgery**
>
> 1. Well circumscribed lesions
> 2. Minimal spinal cord compromise
> 3. Previously irradiated lesions
> 4. Recurrent surgical lesions
> 5. Lesions requiring difficult surgical approaches
> 6. Relatively short life-expectancy as an exclusion criteria for open surgical intervention
> 7. Significant medical comorbidities precluding open surgical intervention
> 8. No overt spinal instability

The ideal lesion should be well circumscribed such that the lesion can be easily outlined for treatment planning. Our initial experience has found that many of our patients harbor lesions that have failed previous treatment modalities such as surgery or external beam irradiation. Many malignant lesions are those that have already been irradiated with significant spinal cord doses or have recurred after open surgical removal. Other candidate lesions are those, either benign or malignant, that would require difficult surgical approaches for complete resection. Candidate patients might have significant medical comorbidities precluding open surgical intervention or a relatively short life-expectancy that would exclude them for open surgical intervention. We have treated several malignant lesions that have completed external beam irradiation with or without IMRT, and we have used CyberKnife radiosurgery for a boost treatment. Other malignant lesions have been treated with CyberKnife radiosurgery as their sole radiation treatment. The benefits for this treatment option include a single treatment with minimal radiation dose to other normal tissue.

If a tumor is only partially resected during an open surgery, fiducials can be left in place to allow for radiosurgery treatment to the residual tumor at a later date. Given the steep fall off gradient of the CyberKnife target dose, such treatments can be given early in the postoperative period as opposed to the usual significant delay before standard external beam irradiation is permitted by the surgeon. Radiation is well known to be effective as a treatment for pain associated with spinal malignancies. We have found CyberKnife spine radiosurgery to be highly effective at decreasing pain in this patient population. Spine radiosurgery was also found to alleviate radicular pain caused by tumor compression.

Unlike conventional radiation therapy that delivers a full dose to both the vertebral body and the spinal cord, the CyberKnife can deliver a single high dose fraction of radiation to the target tissue while sparing most of the adjacent spinal cord. The treatment plan can create a high gradient dose fall off to the target tissue that should significantly reduce the possibility of radiation-induced myelopathy. This is the main advantage to using stereotactic radiosurgery for treatment of spinal tumors.

There are several relative contraindications for CyberKnife spinal radiosurgery. These include: (1) evidence of overt spinal instability, (2) neurologic deficit resulting from bony compression of neural structures, or (3) previous radiation treatment to spinal cord tolerance dose. With time and further clinical experience, these contraindications will be better understood and defined.

Overview of CyberKnife Treatment

The CyberKnife spinal radiosurgery treatment consists of three distinct components: (1) CT image acquisition based upon skull bony landmarks or implanted bone fiducials, (2) treatment planning, and (3) the treatment itself. Intracranial and cervical lesions are tracked relative to skull bony landmarks. All other lesions are tracked relative to fiducials placed adjacent to the lesion. Because these implanted fiducials have a fixed relationship with the bone in which they are implanted, any movement in the tumor in or adjacent to the vertebrae would be detected as movement in the fiducials, and this movement is detected and compensated for by the CyberKnife.

Facemask and Fiducial Placement

All patients with cervical lesions are first fitted with a noninvasive molded Aquaplast facemask (WRF/Aquaplast Corp., Wyckoff, NJ) that stabilizes the head and neck on a radiographically transparent headrest. The patient then proceeds directly with imaging. Computed tomographic (CT) images are acquired using 1.25 mm thick slices from the top of the skull to the bottom of the cervical spine. Images may be acquired using the addition of intravenous contrast enhancement. However, contrast is often not necessary for lesions that are completely within the bony elements. In fact, bony windowing is often more helpful for lesion localization and treatment planning than soft tissue windowing for many spinal lesions. For patients with allergies to intravenous contrast or renal function that precludes contrast, non-enhanced CT imaging is performed with little difficulty in determining precise lesion anatomy.

The CyberKnife is able to detect and track either straight gold fiducials (Alpha-Omega Services, Inc., Bellflower, CA) (Fig. 3) or stainless steel screws (Accuray, Inc., Sunnyvale, CA) (Fig. 4).

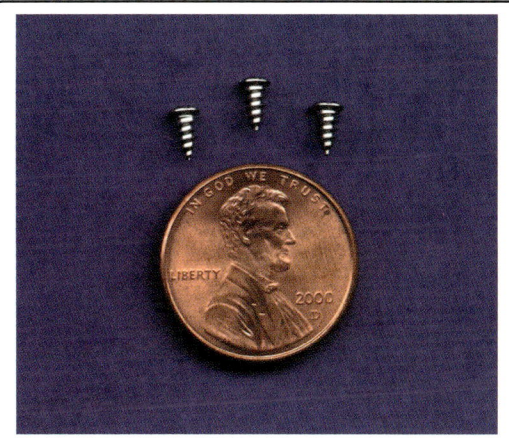

Figure 4. Stainless steel screws used for image tracking.

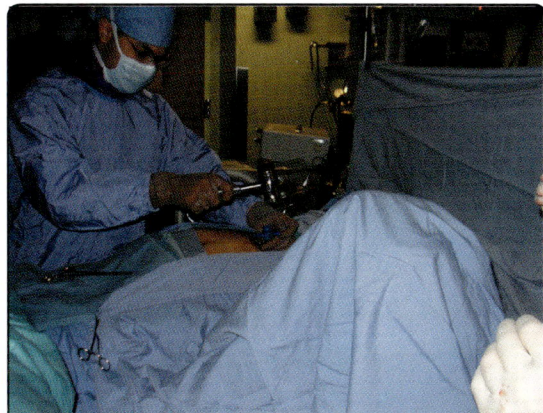

Figure 5. Fiducials are percutaneously placed around the lesion in the bony structures using fluoroscopic guidance.

The fiducial placement procedure is performed in the operating room in an outpatient setting. The gold fiducial markers are placed into the pedicles immediately adjacent to the lesion to be treated using a standard Jamshidi Bone Marrow Biopsy Needle (Allegiance Healthcare Corporation, McGraw Park, IL). The stainless steel screws are screwed directly into the posterior bony elements via a specially designed cannula. If fiducials are placed in conjunction with an open surgical procedure, the stainless steel screws are easily screwed into any adjacent exposed bone.

Four to five fiducial markers are usually placed,

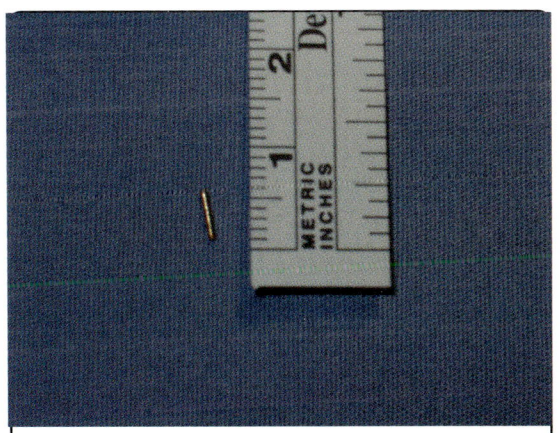

Figure 3. Gold fiducial used for fiducial tracking.

two in the vertebrae above, two in the vertebrae below, and one or two in the vertebrae at the level of the lesion. The reason for this number is that four fiducials are usually tracked during treatment to allow for maximum accuracy. Tracking more than four fiducials adds little to target accuracy. Three fiducials are required to define a full spatial transformation in all six degrees of target translation and rotation. An extra fiducial is placed to allow for a margin of error in case one fiducial cannot be properly imaged or perhaps migrates after placement. Fiducial migration has rarely occurred in our experience.

The fiducials may be placed literally anywhere near or around the target. The principle is that their position must be fixed relative to the target location. For fiducials in the same vertebral body, it is preferable for them to be placed as closely as possible in the same coronal plane so that overlap in an orthogonal projection during X-ray imaging acquisition is minimized (Fig. 6).

For patients with lesions in non-adjacent vertebral bodies, fiducials are sometimes placed between the two lesions. For example, for two lesions at T11 and L3, fiducials may be placed at T12, L1, and L2 without compromising target accuracy.

Treatment Planning

The patient returns as an outpatient for the treatment planning CT. The patient is placed in a supine position in a conformal alpha cradle during CT imaging as well as during treatment. CT images are acquired using 1.25 mm thick slices to include the target lesion as well as all fiducials.

Each radiosurgical treatment plan should be devised jointly by a team comprised of a neurosurgeon, a radiation oncologist, and a radiation physicist. In each case, the radiosurgical treatment plan is designed based on tumor geometry, proximity to spinal cord, and location. Treatment planning is performed using the Accuray treatment planning system DTS 3.0 (Fig. 7A,B). The tumor dose is determined based upon the histology of the tumor, spinal cord tolerance, and previous radiation quantity.

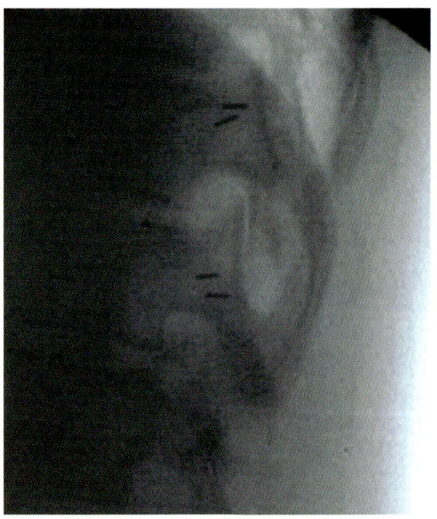

Figure 6. Lateral radiograph of fiducials that have been placed within the pedicles of the thoracic spine. There is a single fiducial within each pedicle. Note that they are in the same coronal plane, thus allowing for maximum distance as seen from an orthogonal position.

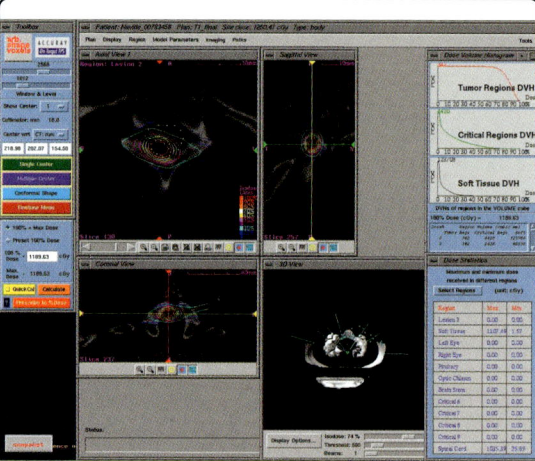

Figure 7(A). The treatment planning screen. A sample treatment plan developed for a thoracic intradural lesion. The 80% isodose represents the prescribed dose of 1250 cGy, the tumor volume is 0.34 cc, and 0.02 cc of the spinal cord received greater than 800 cGy.

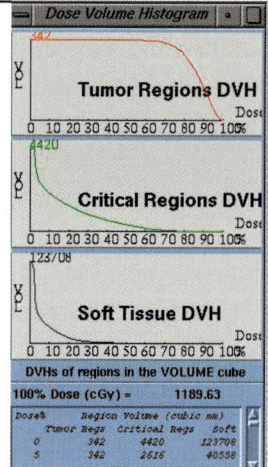

Figure 7(B). The dose volume histogram for the same treatment plan shows that 83.3% of the tumor volume received 80% of the maximum dose of 1250 cGy.

We prescribe the tumor dose to the 80% isodose line. Tumor dose is maintained at 1200-2000 cGy to the 80% isodose line contoured at the edge of the target volume. The maximum intratumoral dose ranges from 1250 to 2500 cGy (mean 1688 cGy). For all cases, the entire spinal canal is treated as the "spinal cord," even for lumbar and sacral lesions.

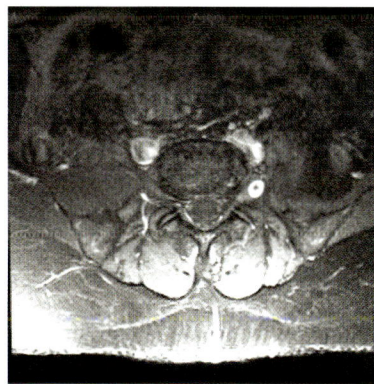

Figure 8(A). Gadolinium-enhanced MR image of a left L5 neurofibroma in a patient with Neurofibromatosis and severe left L5 radicular pain.

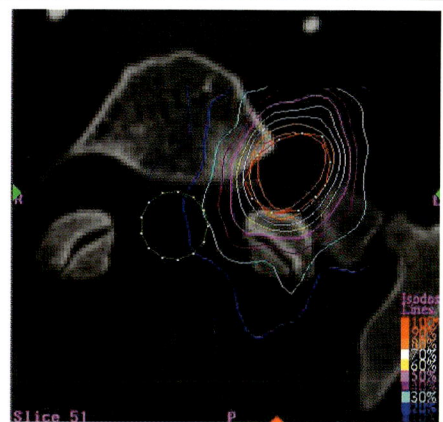

Figure 8(B). The left L5 neurofibroma target. 80% isodose line represents prescribed dose of 2000 cGy. The lesion volume was 3.2 cc. The maximum dose to the thecal sac was 660 cGy. The patient had excellent pain relief within 1 month that has lasted for one year.

A limit of 800 cGy is set as the maximum spinal cord dose for treatment planning calculations. The spinal cord volume receiving greater than 800 cGy ranges from 0.0 to 1.3 cc (mean 0.3 cc). A limit of 200 cGy is set as the maximal dose to each of the kidneys.

In our experience, the mean tumor volume is approximately 30 cc (range, 0.3 to 168 cc). This is approximately ten times the average volume of intracranial lesions treated by radiosurgery. The lesion is outlined based upon CT imaging. An "inverse treatment planning" technique is always utilized such that the tumor receives the maximum dose allowable as restricted by the maximum spinal cord tolerance dose, as well as other critical structures such as small bowel and kidneys.

Dose Prescriptions

There is no large experience to date with spinal radiosurgery that has previously developed optimal doses for this treatment technique. The dose to the tumor margin is based on tumor histology, location, and history of prior fractionated radiotherapy. Records regarding previous spinal cord irradiation are carefully considered. Many lesions have received prior external beam irradiation with maximum spinal cord doses. Published reports from the Stanford CyberKnife experience indicate that spinal lesions received total treatment doses of 1100 to 2500 cGy in one to five fractions (3). We have delivered total treatment doses of 1200 to 2200 cGy to the 80% isodose line (Fig. 9).

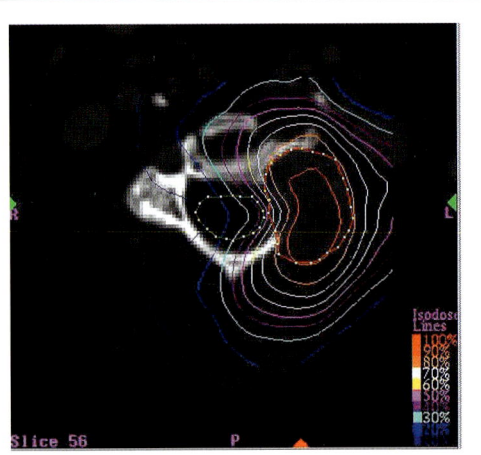

Figure 9. Renal cell metastasis to the C5 lateral mass. The patient had severe pain that recurred after external beam irradiation. The tumor was treated with 14 Gy to the 80% isodose. Note the conformality of the isodose line around the spinal cord.

All of these were delivered in a single fraction. The higher doses were for lesions away from critical structures. This translated into a maximum tumor dose (measured at the center of the target) of 1500 to 2500 cGy.

There is little experience regarding the tolerance of the human spinal cord to single fraction doses. In a review evaluating 172 patients treated with fractionated radiotherapy to the cervical and thoracic spine at the University of California, San Francisco (total dose of 4000 to 7000 cGy fractionated over a 2 to 3 week period), Wara et al. (26) reported nine cases of radiation-induced myelopathy. Three out of nine patients had mild cervical cord neurological deficits without any significant long-term symptoms. The length of the spinal cord that was exposed to radiation averaged from 4 to 22 cm. Hatlevoll et al. (27) reported a series of 387 patients with bronchial carcinoma treated with a split-course regimen using large single fractions. Seventeen patients developed radiation myelitis with average total dose of 3800 cGy. Kim et al. (28) reported 7 patients with transverse myelopathy from a group of 109 patients treated with definitive radiotherapy for head and neck cancers to a total dose of 5700 to 6200 cGy with an average field size of 10 by 10 cm. Abbatucci et al. (29) reported 8/203 cases of radiation-induced myelopathy with a total radiation dose of 5400 to 6000 cGy to the cervical and thoracic spine. McCunniff et al. (30) reported only 1 case of radiation myelopathy out of 652 patients who had received greater than 6,000 cGy using standard fractionation. Phillips et al. (31) reported 3 cases of transverse myelitis in 350 patients with tumors to the chest treated to a total radiation dose of 3300 to 4350 cGy. Based upon this literature review, the incidence of radiation induced myelopathy using conventionally fractionated radiotherapy to the cervical and thoracic spine ranged from 0.2% to 5%.

We use 800 cGy as the maximum allowable dose to the spinal cord during inverse treatment planning. We limit each kidney dose to 200 cGy. This especially becomes important in the treatment of lower thoracic and lumbar vertebrae, even more so if the patient has undergone a nephrectomy or received nephrotoxic chemotherapy.

Treatment Delivery

The third component of the CyberKnife treatment is the actual treatment delivery. Treatments may be performed using either a single or multiple fractions in an outpatient setting. We prefer a single fraction technique. The patients are placed on the CyberKnife treatment couch in a supine position with the appropriate immobilization device (Fig. 10).

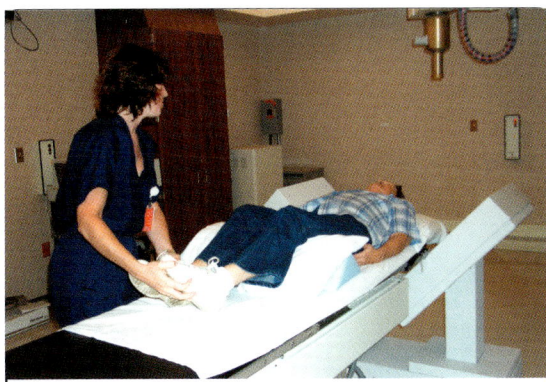

Figure 10. Patient setup on the CyberKnife treatment couch. The patient is positioned supine with legs in an alpha cradle for comfort and to limit motion. The couch will move rostrally to place the fiducials between the amorphous silicon detectors.

Some patients with thoracic or lumbar lesions localized with fiducials are actually more comfortable without the alpha cradle, and only pillows are used. During the treatment, real time digital x-ray images of the patient are obtained in order to track either skull bony landmarks or implanted fiducials (Fig. 11).

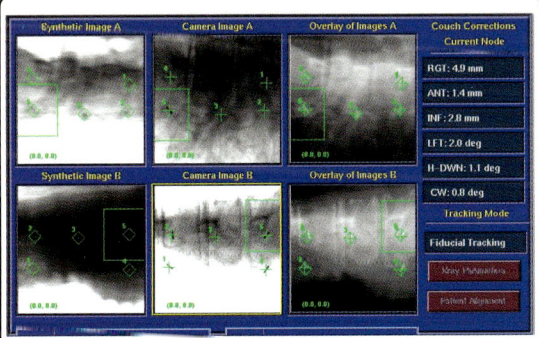

Figure 11. All five fiducials are tracked for thoracic and lumbar lesions using real-time image guidance. The measured position as seen by both cameras is communicated through a real-time control loop to a robotic manipulator that redirects the beam to the precise intended target.

The location of the vertebral body being treated is established from these images and is used to determine tumor location as previously described.

The patient is observed throughout the treatment by closed circuit television. No pulse oximetry or other monitoring is used during the treatment. The patient is asked to wave their hand or speak if they would like to temporarily halt the treatment. The duration of the treatment is approximately one to two hours. Many of these patients are in significant pain and are uncomfortable in the supine position for prolonged periods of time. No intravenous sedation is used, only oral analgesics. It is very easy to pause the treatment at any time for the patient to sit up. After a brief rest, the patient returns to the supine position on the treatment couch and the treatment resumes. Mild, transient nausea may be experienced by patients receiving treatment to lumbar lesions. For these cases, patients are pretreated with anti-emetics.

Summary

Tumors of the spine affect a large number of patients each year, resulting in significant pain, destruction of the spinal column causing mechanical instability, and neurological deficits. Standard therapeutic options include surgery and fractionated external beam radiotherapy. The first option can be associated with significant morbidity and limited local tumor control. Radiotherapy may provide less than optimal pain relief since the total dose is limited by the tolerance of adjacent tissues (e.g. spinal cord). Therefore, improved treatment would be beneficial in providing a better quality of life. The proposed treatment represents a logical extension of the current state-of-the-art radiation therapy. It has the potential to significantly improve local control of cancer of the spine, which could translate into more effective palliation. Another advantage to the patient is that irradiation can be completed in a single day rather than several weeks, which is not inconsequential for patients with a limited life expectancy. In addition, cancer patients may have difficulty with access to a radiation treatment facility for prolonged, daily fractionated therapy. Finally, the procedure is minimally invasive and can be performed in an outpatient setting.

Stereotactic radiosurgery now has a feasible and safe delivery system available for the treatment of spinal lesions. The major potential benefit of radiosurgical ablation of spinal lesions is relatively short treatment time in an outpatient setting combined with potentially better local control of the tumor with minimal risk of side effects. Such an outcome could translate into better palliation of symptoms and longer survival period. In addition, this technique will allow for the treatment of lesions previously irradiated using external beam radiation. This new technique offers an alternative therapeutic modality for the treatment of spinal neoplasms in medically inoperable patients, previously irradiated sites, and for lesions not amenable to open surgical techniques or as an adjunct to surgery.

References

1 Gerszten PC, Welch WC. Current surgical management of metastatic spinal disease. *Oncology* 2000; 14; 1013-24.

2 Faul CM, Flickinger JC. The use of radiation in the management of spinal metastases. *J Neurooncol* 1995; 23; 149-61.

3 Ryu SI, Chang SD, Kim DH et al. Image-guided Hypo-fractionated Stereotactic Radiosurgery to Spinal Lesions. *Neurosurgery* 2001; 49; 838 - 46.

4 Loblaw DA, Laperriere NJ. Emergency Treatment of Malignant Extradural Spinal Cord Compression: An Evidence-Based Guideline. *Journal of Clinical Oncology* 1998; 16; 1613-24.

5 Colombo F, Benedetti A, Pozza F et al. Stereotactic Radiosurgery utilizing a linear accelerator. *Appl Neurophysiol* 1985; 48; 133-45.

6 Hitchcock E, Kitchen G, Dalton E et al. Stereotactic linac radiosurgery. *British J of Neurosurgery* 1989; 3; 305-12.

7 Milker-Zabel S, Zabel A, Thilmann C et al. Clinical Results of Retreatment of Vertebral Bone Metastases by Stereotactic Conformal Radiotherapy and Intensity-Modulated Radiotherapy. *Int J Rad Onc Biol Phys* 2003; 55; 162-7.

8 Hamilton AJ, Lulu BL, Fosmire H et al. Preliminary clinical experience with linear accelerator-based spinal stereotactic radiosurgery. *Neurosurgery* 1995; 36; 311-9.

9 Kuriyama K, Onishi H, Sano N et al. A New Irradiation Unit Constructed of Self-Moving Gantry-CT and Linac. *Int J Rad Onc Biol Phys* 2003; 55; 428-35.

10 Alexander E, Loeffler JS, Lunsford LD. *Stereotactic Radiosurgery.* New York: McGraw-Hill, Inc, 1993.

11 Kaplan ID, Adler JR, Hicks WLJ et al. Radiosurgery for palliation of base of skull recurrences from head and neck cancers. *Cancer* 1992; 10; 1-16.

12 Loeffler JS, Kooy HM, Wen PY et al. The treatment of recurrent brain metastases with stereotactic radiosurgery. *J Clinical Oncology* 1990; 8; 576-82.

13 Steiner L, Lindquist C, Adler JR et al. Clinical outcome of radiosurgery for cerebral arteriovenous malformations. *J Neurosurg* 1992; 77; 1-8.

14 Lunsford LD, Flickinger JC, Coffey RJ. Stereotactic gamma knife radiosurgery. Initial North American experience in 207 patients. *Arch Neurol* 1990; 47; 169-75.

15 Adler JR, Chang SD, Murphy MJ et al. The CyberKnife: A frameless robotic system for radiosurgery. *Stereotactic and Functional Neurosurgery* 1997; 60; 124-8.

16 Adler JR, Murphy MJ, Chang SD et al. Image-guided robotic radiosurgery. *Neurosurgery* 1999; 44; 1299-307.

17 Gerszten P, Ozhasoglu C, Burton S et al. Feasibility of frameless single-fraction stereotactic radiosurgery for spinal lesions. *Neurosurgery Focus* 2002; 13; 1-6.

18 Murphy MJ, Chang S, Gibbs I et al. Image-guided radiosurgery in the treatment of spinal metastases. *Neurosurg Focus* 2001; 11; 1-7.

19 Chang SD, Adler JR. Current status and optimal use of radiosurgery. *Oncology* 2001; 209-21.

20 Adler JR, Murphy MJ, Chang SD et al. Image-guided robotic radiosurgery. *Neurosurgery* 1999; 44; 1-8.

21 Adler JR, Cox RS, Kaplan I et al. Stereotactic radiosurgical treatment of brain metastases. *J Neurosurg* 1992; 76; 444-9.

22 Guthrie BL, Adler JR. Computer-assisted preoperative planning, interactive surgery, and frameless stereotaxy. *Clinical Neurosurgery* 1991; 38; 112-31.

11 Kaplan ID, Adler JR, Hicks WLJ et al. Radiosurgery for palliation of base of skull recurrences from head and neck cancers. *Cancer* 1992; 10; 1-16.

12 Loeffler JS, Kooy HM, Wen PY et al. The treatment of recurrent brain metastases with stereotactic radiosurgery. *J Clinical Oncology* 1990; 8; 576-82.

13 Steiner L, Lindquist C, Adler JR et al. Clinical outcome of radiosurgery for cerebral arteriovenous malformations. *J Neurosurg* 1992; 77; 1-8.

14 Lunsford LD, Flickinger JC, Coffey RJ. Stereotactic gamma knife radiosurgery. Initial North American experience in 207 patients. *Arch Neurol* 1990; 47; 169-75.

15 Adler JR, Chang SD, Murphy MJ et al. The CyberKnife: A frameless robotic system for radiosurgery. *Stereotactic and Functional Neurosurgery* 1997; 60; 124-8.

16 Adler JR, Murphy MJ, Chang SD et al. Image-guided robotic radiosurgery. *Neurosurgery* 1999; 44; 1299-307.

17 Gerszten P, Ozhasoglu C, Burton S et al. Feasibility of frameless single-fraction stereotactic radiosurgery for spinal lesions. *Neurosurgery Focus* 2002; 13; 1-6.

18 Murphy MJ, Chang S, Gibbs I et al. Image-guided radiosurgery in the treatment of spinal metastases. *Neurosurg Focus* 2001; 11; 1-7.

19 Chang SD, Adler JR. Current status and optimal use of radiosurgery. *Oncology* 2001; 209-21.

20 Adler JR, Murphy MJ, Chang SD et al. Image-guided robotic radiosurgery. *Neurosurgery* 1999; 44; 1-8.

21 Adler JR, Cox RS, Kaplan I et al. Stereotactic radiosurgical treatment of brain metastases. *J Neurosurg* 1992; 76; 444-9.

22 Guthrie BL, Adler JR. Computer-assisted preoperative planning, interactive surgery, and frameless stereotaxy. *Clinical Neurosurgery* 1991; 38; 112-31.

23 Murphy MJ, Cox RS. The accuracy of dose localization for an image-guided frameless radiosurgery system. *Medical Physics* 1996; 23; 2043-9.

24 Murphy MJ, Cox RS. Frameless Radiosurgery using real-time image correlation for beam targeting. *Medical Physics* 1996; 23; 1052-3.

25 Chang SD, Main W, Martin DP et al. An Analysis of The Accuracy of the CyberKnife: A Robotic Frameless Stereotactic Radiosurgical System. *Neurosurgery* 2003; 52; 140-7.

26 Wara WM, Phillips TL, Sheline GE et al. Radiation tolerance of the spinal cord. *Cancer* 1975; 35; 1558-62.

27 Hatlevoll R, Host H, Kaalhus O. Myelopathy following radiotherapy of bronchial carcinoma with large single fractions: A retrospective study. *Int J Radiat Oncol Biol Phys* 1983; 9; 41-4.

28 Kim YH, Fayos JV. Radiation tolerance of the cervical spinal cord. *Radiology 1981*; 2:139; 473-8.

29 Abbatucci JS, Delozier T, Quint R et al. Radiation myelopathy of the cervical spinal cord: time, dose and volume factors. *Int J Radiat Oncol Biol Phys* 1978; 4; 239-48.

30 McCuniff AJ, Liang MJ. Radiation tolerance of the cervical spinal cord. *Int J Radiat Oncol Biol Phys* 1989; 16; 675-8.

31 Phillips TL, Buschke F. Radiation tolerance of the thoracic spinal cord. *AJR* 1969; 105; 659-64.

The authors note that a modifed version of this chapter has been submitted to Techniques in Neurosurgery.

CyberKnife Radiosurgery for Trigeminal Neuralgia

Pantaleo Romanelli
Steven D. Chang
Gary Heit

Introduction

Gamma Knife Radiosurgery (GKR) is an effective minimally-invasive therapeutic option for trigeminal neuralgia (TN). GKR is commonly offered to patients who have failed to respond to other procedures or who are poor surgical candidates because of age or concomitant medical problems. The relatively low incidence of side effects (mostly related to reduced facial sensory function) is associated with pain outcomes comparable to those offered by more invasive treatments. The median time to achieve more than 50% pain relief was about two months in one of the largest series published (1). For this reason, patients requiring immediate pain relief are rarely treated with GKR. Immediate pain relief can be achieved by means of invasive treatments including microvascular decompression, radiofrequency rhizotomy and balloon compression. A much shorter delay for the development of analgesia has been appreciated in a small cohort of patients undergoing CyberKnife radiosurgery for TN. The CyberKnife exploits the highly maneuverable robotic arm of an image-guided LINAC to deliver conformal irradiation without a rigid frame. A combination of factors including improved targeting accuracy due to CT-ventriculography, improved treatment planning due to the absence of the stereotactic ring, conformal irradiation and treatment of an extended length of the nerve could be responsible for such an early response.

Patient Selection

CyberKnife radiosurgery is offered to medically-refractory TN patients that have failed or refuse surgery or are not suitable candidates for invasive intervention due to age or medical contrainidications to surgery.

CT Cisternography

To obtain an accurate distortion-free localization of the trigeminal nerve, CT cisternography is performed. This technique produces excellent visualization of the structures contained in the posterior fossa, especially the cranial nerves (2). Five cc's of Omnipaque-300 are instilled in the thecal sac by lumbar puncture. The patient is kept in the Trendelenburg position for about 30 minutes to facilitate the diffusion of the contrast in the basal cisterns. A thin section CT scan (175 slices, thickness: 1.25 mm) is made through the entire head, showing the anatomy of the basal cisterns and outlining the entire length of the trigeminal nerve from its origin in the brainstem to its entry into the Meckel's cave. (Figure 1)

Treatment Planning and Delivery

The CT images are networked to the CyberKnife work station where the trigeminal nerve is outlined. The most proximal point of the nerve identified for purposes of treatment planning is 3 mm

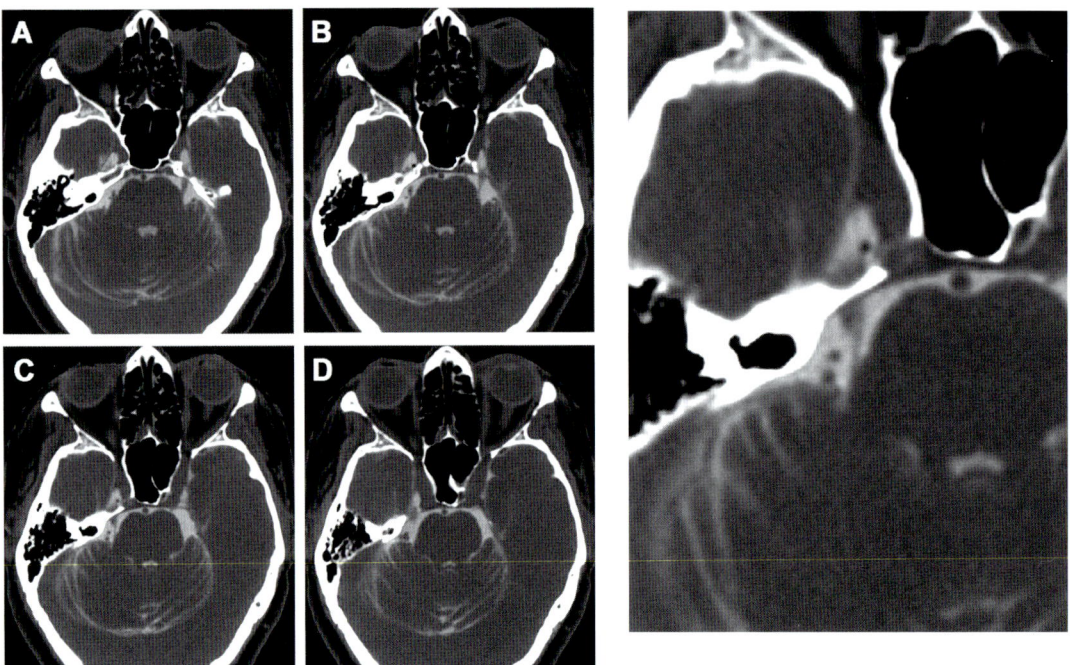

Figure 1 and 2. CT-cisternography showing well defined trigeminal nerve.

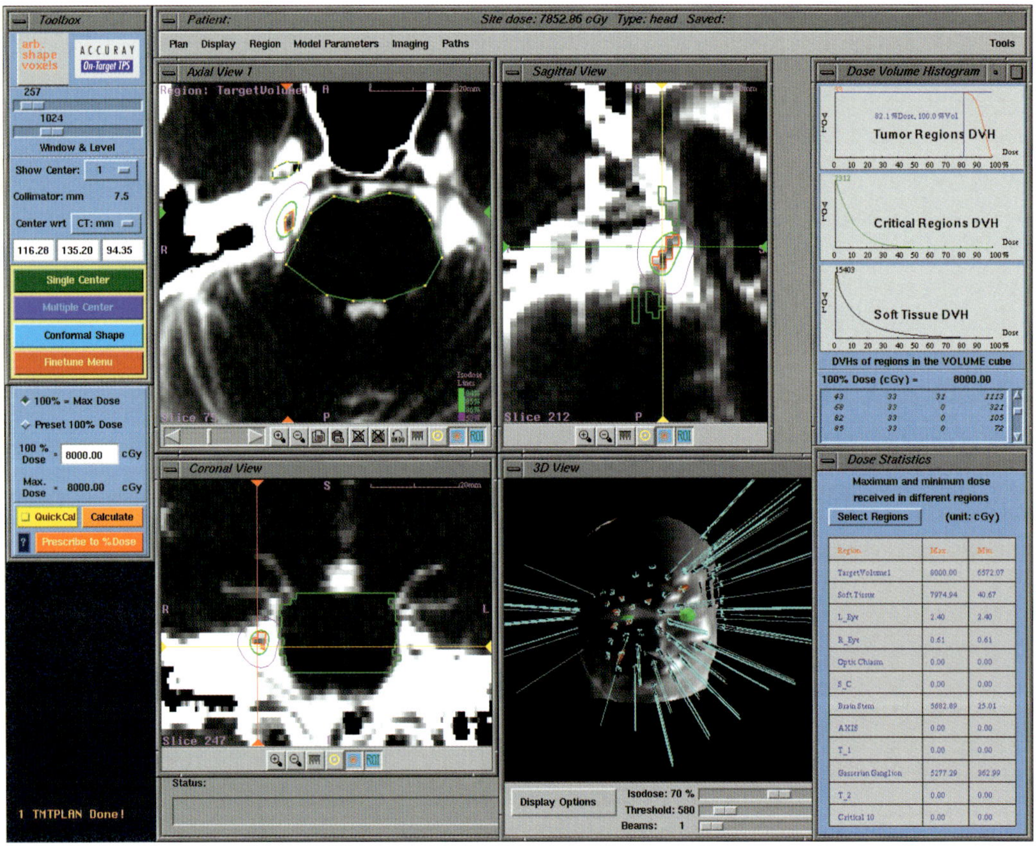

Figure 3. Treatment plan for TN radiosurgery

away from the brain stem. The total length of the nerve outlined is typically 8 mm. The 80% isodose line is then prescribed, encompassing approximately 8 mm of the nerve from a point 3 mm away from the root entry zone to the area where the nerve leaves the intracranial space to enter into the Meckel's cave (Figure 2). This treatment volume receives a conformal irradiation delivering an approximate average of 64 Gy to the prescribed 80% isodose line. The treatment conformality is produced by the robot's six-degree-of-freedom maneuverability that allows an array of overlapping beams to be superimposed without an isocenter. The inverse planning procedure optimizes the set of beam directions, delivering a more homogeneous dose distribution that closely conforms to the trigeminal nerve as compared to that achieved by frame-based systems.

Image-Guided Radiosurgery

A compact 6 MV X-ray LINAC is accurately positioned by a robotic arm that can move and point the LINAC with six degrees of freedom (3, 4). Two x-ray imaging devices based on amorphous silicon detectors are positioned on either side of the patient's anatomy and acquire real-time digital radiographs of the skull at repeated intervals during treatment. The images are automatically registered to digitally reconstructed radiographs derived from the treatment planning CT. This registration process allows the position of the skull (and thus the treatment site) to be translated to the coordinate frame of the LINAC. A control loop between the imaging system and the robotic arm adjusts the pointing of the LINAC therapeutic beam to the observed position of the treatment anatomy (target). If the patient moves, the change is detected during the next imaging cycle and the beam is adjusted and realigned with the target.

Dose Placement Precision

The most important performance characteristic of the CyberKnife is the accuracy with which it can place the dose distribution. Application accuracy for the CyberKnife radiosurgery system is based on the accuracy of beam delivery, which combines the robot and the camera image system tracking system, and the accuracy of target localization, which combines computed tomographic (CT) imaging and treatment planning (5, 6).

Results

Seventeen patients with idiopathic TN were treated with CyberKnife radiosurgery. CT cisternography was obtained in fifteen, producing an excellent visualization of the trigeminal nerve in all, except for one patient with an atrophic nerve. The treatment planning was greatly enhanced by the accurate imaging of the trigeminal nerve produced by CT cisternography. In particular, it was possible to target an extended length of the nerve (average: 7.4 mm; range: 5-10 mm). Mean target volume was 0.065 cc (range: 0.033- 0.158 cc). An average 82.5% isodose line (range: 79-87) was used to deliver a mean prescribed dose of 65.4 Gy (range: 60-70 Gy). The mean maximum dose was 79.2 Gy (range: 72.3-86.4 Gy). Mean follow-up was 7.3 months (range: 1-15 months).

Clinical Outcomes

Fifteen out of seventeen patients (88.2 %) developed satisfactory pain relief after radiosurgery. One patient with atypical features relapsed after six months of pain relief while another patient developed bothersome paresthesias two months after the treatment. Overall, 13 patients out of 17 (76.5 %) have achieved and maintained a good outcome after an average follow-up of 7.3 months. Six of these 13 patients are now off medications while the other seven patients are in the process to be tapered off.

Temporal Patterns of Pain Relief

The latency of complete pain relief was approximately one day in five patients, one week in four, one month in three, two months in one and six months in two. Out of fifteen patients developing a satisfactory therapeutic response, nine (60%) achieved pain relief within one week. These nine patients received a prescribed dose of 66 Gy or more. Lower prescribed doses were associated with a progressively increasing latency to pain relief.

Side Effects Related to Radiosurgery

Four patients experiencing immediate pain relief developed facial hypoesthesia. They received 66 to 70 Gy to an isodose ranging from 79 to 82% and a maximum dose ranging from 80 to 86.4 Gy. One case of corneal numbness was detected approximately 6 months after the treatment in a patient who received 60 Gy to the 83% isodose and a maximum dose of 72.3 Gy.

Discussion

TN patients treated with CyberKnife radiosurgery can develop pain relief with a substantially shorter latency in comparison to patients undergoing TN GKR. Patients treated with GKR usually develop analgesia after a latency period of 2 to 6 months (1, 7, 8, 9, 10, 11, 12). Obviously, the small number of CyberKnife patients presented here does not allow us to consider this data anything more than preliminary. There are several possible explanations for the fast onset of pain relief after CyberKnife radiosurgery. First, the targeting technique based on positive contrast CT cisternography could be more accurate than conventional MR-based targeting, due to the lack of image distortion. Second, the absence of the frame avoids any restriction to the treatment planning and to the delivery of radiation. Third, the conformal delivery of radiation allows the homogeneous irradiation of an expanded length of the nerve. Probably a combination of these factors is responsible for a more thorough irradiation of the nerve. Clinically relevant accuracy of the CyberKnife radiosurgery system is based on the beam delivery accuracy, which combines the robot and the camera image tracking system, and the target localization accuracy, which combines CT imaging and treatment planning. A phantom study found that mean errors of the second generation CyberKnife currently in use at Stanford University Medical Center ranged from 0.7 mm for a CT slice thickness of 0.625 mm to 1.97 mm for a CT slice thickness of 3.75 mm (Chang). An average radial error of 1.14 mm (SD: 0.3 mm) was found using a CT slice thickness of 1.25 mm. CT-based positive contrast identification of the trigeminal nerve using 1.25 mm slices helps to outline and target the entire length of the nerve, sparing the proximal 3 mm to reduce the brain stem irradiation. In contrast, MR-based stereotactic systems can produce an average localization error of 5 mm (13).

An additional factor improving the radiation delivery to the nerve is the treatment conformality of CyberKnife radiosurgery. A fixed isocenter, where all beams converge on a well defined point, is the basis for standard radiosurgery instruments such as the Gamma Knife and conventional linear accelerators. This concept works well with spherical targets but is not ideal for complex or irregular shapes. To treat non-spherical targets, isocentric radiosurgical methods rely on multiple overlapping spherical dose volumes, a method which results in target dose heterogeneity. The elongated shape of the trigeminal nerve is suboptimally treated by a single spherical irradiation and may require repeated irradiation using a second isocenter, usually located more anteriorly along the nerve. This approach may produce increased morbidity (14). The conformal irradiation provided by the CyberKnife is especially convenient for the treatment of an elongated structure such as the TN because there is a homogeneous irradiation of the target, and also an extensive length of the nerve can be treated.

In our series, patients who received a prescribed dose of 66 Gy or higher developed satisfactory pain relief within one week. Patients who received lower doses developed pain relief approximately 1 to 6 months after the treatment. It should be stressed that a longer follow-up period is necessary before definitive statements about the efficacy of CyberKnife radiosurgery for TN can be made. For example, the onset of corneal anesthesia six months after the delivery of a 60 Gy prescribed dose (maximum dose: 72.3 Gy) suggests that delayed complications may occur even with lower doses.

Conclusion

CyberKnife radiosurgery is able to produce early immediate pain relief in patients with trigeminal neuralgia. Larger patient samples are necessary to validate these findings. A combination of conformal irradiation and increased targeting accuracy due to CT cisternography could explain this interesting phenomenon. An optimal dose range able to produce pain relief while minimizing facial sensory denervation needs to be established.

References

1. Kondziolka D, Dade Lunsford L, Flickinger JC. Stereotactic radiosurgery for the treatment of Trigeminal Neuralgia. Clin J Pain, 18: 42-47, 2002
2. Mawad ME, Silver AJ, Hilal SK, et al: Computed tomography of the brain stem with intrathecal Metrizamide. Part I: The normal brain stem. AJR140:553–563, 1983
3. Adler JR, Jr., Murphy MJ, Chang SD, et al. Image-guided robotic radiosurgery. Neurosurgery. 1999; 44:1299-306; discussion 306-7.
4. Murphy MJ. An automatic six-degree-of-freedom image registration algorithm for image-guided frameless stereotaxic radiosurgery. Med Phys 1997; 24:857-866
5. Murphy MJ, Cox RS. The accuracy of dose localization for an image-guided frameless radiosurgery system. Med Phys.1996; 23:2043-9.
6. Chang SD, Main W., Martin D.P., et al. An analysis of the accuracy of the CyberKnife: A robotic frameless stereotactic radiosurgical system. Neurosurgery. 2003; 52:140-147
7. Kondziolka D, Lunsford LD, Flickinger JC, et al: Stereotactic radiosurgery for trigeminal neuralgia: a multiinstitutional study using the gamma unit. J Neurosurg 84:940–945, 1996
8. Rand RW: Leksell gamma knife treatment of tic douloureux. Neurosurg Clin North Am 8:75–78, 1997
9. Urgosik D, Vymazal J, Vladyka V, et al: Gamma knife treatment of trigeminal neuralgia: clinical and electrophysiological study. Stereotact Funct Neurosurg 70 (suppl 1):200–109, 1998
10. Young RF: Functional neurosurgery with the Leksell gamma knife. Stereotact Funct Neurosurg 66:19–23, 1996
11. Regis J, Bartolomei F, Metellus P, Rey M, Genton P, Dravet C, Bureau M, Semah H, Gastaut JL, Peragut JC, Chauvel P : Radiosurgery for trigeminal neuralgia and epilepsy. Neurosurg Clin N Am 10;359-377,1999
12. Young RF, Jacques DS, Mark R, Vermculen S, Coputt B, Li F: Gamma knife treatment of trigeminal neuralgia: long-term experience. Proceedings of the 10th International Meeting of the Leksell Gamma Knife Society, 2000 (abstract).
13. Heilbrun MP: Image-guided stereotactic surgery: Adjunct technical advances, in Wilkins RH, Rengachary SS(eds): Neurosurgery Update II. New York: McGraw-Hill, 1991, pp 373-378.
14. Pollock BE, Phuong LK, Foote RL, Stafford SL, Gorman DA. High-dose trigeminal neuralgia radiosurgery associated with increased risk of trigeminal nerve dysfunction. Neurosurgery 49: 58-64,2001

Radiobiology and Radiosurgery

Iris C. Gibbs

Shortly after Roentgen discovered x-rays in 1895 and the Curies discovered radium in 1898, the biological effects of radiation were recognized. However, it was not until 1922 that clinical evidence was presented showing that fractionated radiation could cure laryngeal cancer without significant sequelae. Pioneered by the French, this fractioned approach to radiotherapy remains the foundation of radiotherapy today (1).

Though the initial premise of radiation fractionation has its roots in clinical observations, the field of radiobiology in the early part of the 20th century was able to clarify the scientific basis of the clinical observation that some normal tissues were spared irreversible radiation injury if the radiation dose was given as smaller increments over a period of time. In vitro and in vivo studies helped to quantify these observations and helped to determine that DNA was the target for lethal radiation injury. Survival of mammalian cells following exposure to radiation is described by the cell survival curve. (Figure 1.1)

These curves are generated by compiling the data from experiments exposing a population of cells to incremental doses of radiation and counting the number of surviving cells. The surviving fraction of cells is plotted against the dose on a logarithmic scale.

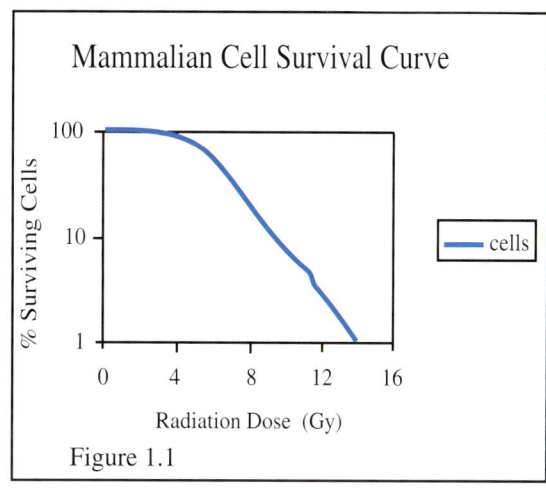

Figure 1.1

The survival curve of mammalian cells exhibits an initial shoulder which represents the accumulation of cells that experience injury without dying, i.e., "sublethal damage." Cells differ in their rates of sublethal damage repair. These differences are shown as differences in the size of the shoulder region of the survival curve based on cell type. Some cells respond early to radiation exposure, the so-called "early-responding tissue," while others respond late, the so-called "late-responding tissue" (1).

The Four R's of Radiobiology

Understanding of tissue response to radiation has led to basic principles of radiotherapy, called the four R's of radiation biology. These are as follows:

1) Re-oxygenation, 2) Repair, 3) Reassortment, 4) Repopulation (2). These principles provide the rationale for various radiation treatment regimens and the premise for radiation fractionation.

Reoxygenation

The presence of oxygen tends to enhance the effect of ionizing radiation on cell kill. This effect is most likely due to radiation-induced free radical production. Tumors contain a mixture of oxygen-rich cells (aerated cells) and oxygen-poor cells (hypoxic cells). Hypoxic cells tend to be more resistant to radiation killing. When a dose of radiation is given, the aerated cells are killed preferentially. The oxygen status of the tumor is not static, but dynamic. Once radiation has killed a proportion of the well-aerated cells, a proportion of the previously hypoxic cells then becomes better oxygenated, and thus more susceptible to radiation killing. This process is known as reoxygenation.

Repair

Cellular repair of radiation damage can occur if the damage itself is not lethal to the cell. The repair of sublethal damage allows cells to tolerate higher total doses of radiation if given in multiple small increments. Cells vary in their capacity to repair. Cells that repair damage slowly, "late responding tissue" (e.g., spinal cord) are spared more by delivering radiation in multiple small fractions as compared to rapidly responding tissue such as bone marrow or mucosa.

Reassortment

Cells increase in number by undergoing a cell division process. In this process, a series of cellular events (phases) occurs in the nucleus and cytoplasm. These phases are M (mitosis), G1 (Gap 1), S (DNA synthesis), G2 (Gap 2). It has been shown that the cell is most sensitive to radiation killing if it is in the M and G2 phases of the cell cycle; and least sensitive in the S and G1 phases. After a dose of radiation, the sensitive cells are killed, leaving mainly the resistant cells behind. If the cells are allowed to continue their propagation through the cell cycle, a proportion will move from a more resistant phase to a sensitive one in a process known as reassortment.

Repopulation

During a course of fractionated radiotherapy, cells in both the tumor and normal tissues continue to undergo cell division. As a response to the radiation, new growth can occur more quickly by shortening the cell cycle or recruiting stem cells. For certain types of tumors, accelerated repopulation of tumor cells may cause the later doses of radiation to be less effective than earlier doses. For this reason, it generally best to avoid protracted courses of radiation (1, 2).

Concept of Radiation Fractionation

Since the effects of radiation are experienced by the target (tumor) tissue as well as normal tissue, the goal of radiation treatment is to maximize killing of the tumor while minimizing the effects on normal tissue. The therapeutic ratio is determined by the maximal separation between curves of dose effects on tumor killing from the curve of normal tissue complications. Based on the four principles set out above, delivery of radiation in small increments separate in time, a technique known as radiation fractionation, appears to satisfy these constraints. Radiation fractionation spares normal tissue by allowing for repair of sublethal damage and repopulation of cells between fractions. It also allows for more tumor killing by reoxygenation of hypoxic cells and reassortment of cells into sensitive phases of the cell cycle.

Fractionation Schemes

A variety of radiation fractionation schemes has been designed in order to best balance the importance of the four principles of radiation for each tumor type. Common fractionation schemes are 1) *conventional fractionation*, 2) *hyperfractionation*, 3) *accelerated fractionation*, and 4) *hypofractionation*.

Conventional fractionation is the delivery of single daily radiation doses of 1.8 - 2 Gy for 5 days a week. Though this regimen was largely developed based on convenience and empirical observations, it remains a standard radiation therapy approach.

Hyperfractionation involves delivering a larger number of less than conventional sized doses of radiation to a higher overall dose. The treatments are generally given to doses of 1.0 - 1.2 Gy several times per day. The hyperfractionation regimen is designed to reduce the risk of complications due to late responding normal tissue effects, which are generally dominated by the fraction size. With *accelerated fractionation* the goal is to reduce the overall treatment time by delivering multiple daily fractions and thereby avoid some adverse effects of tumor repopulation. *Hypofractionation* involves the delivery of a smaller number of larger fractions. The total dose of this regimen is generally lower than that of conventional fractionation in order to reduce the potential for radiation complications.

The alpha-to-beta ratio (α/β)

Formulae have been derived from the concepts of the linear-quadratic model of the cell survival curves to estimate biologically equivalent doses between fractionation regimens.

$$BED = nd\left(1 + \frac{d}{\alpha/\beta}\right)$$

In the linear-quadratic model of cell survival following radiation exposure, there are two components of cell kill, the α component, which represents the initial linear portion of the survival curve, and the β component, which represents the quadratic portion of the curve. The ratio of α/β provides an indication of the cell's sensitivity to radiation exposure. Higher α/β ratios are possessed by cells types, which are more radiosensitive, while cells with lower α/β are more radioresistant.

Tissue Tolerance to Radiation Exposure

Tissue tolerance dose is conventionally defined as that dose which produces an acceptable probability of a treatment complication (3). In the early days of clinical radiation therapy, radiation treatment was limited by the sensitivity of the skin. With the advent of multi-beam treatment, higher energy x-rays, and improved radiation precision, the ability to deliver more effective doses to tumors without causing severe skin necrosis has been possible. The concept of tolerance is essentially one of probability and includes both subjective and objective criteria.

Tolerance Dose

Concept of $TD_{5/5}$ and $TD_{50/5}$

In the late 1960's, Rubin and Casarett introduced a quantitative measure of radiation tolerance using the probabilities $TD_{5/5}$ and $TD_{50/5}$ (4). These terms, $TD_{5/5}$ and $TD_{50/5}$, refer to the probability of developing an objective complication of 5% and 50%, respectively within five years. These values were accepted as estimates of the minimal and maximal dose tolerance, respectively, to optimize tumor control and minimize complications. Since most of the concepts of radiation tolerance were largely based on observations of whole organ tolerance, radiation volume effects were largely ignored until the advent of more conformal radiation therapy techniques. In 1991, a radiation task force was formed to estimate the tolerance of radiation to partial organ volumes (3). These estimates were generated from published reports of clinical observations. Table 1.1 below illustrates a portion of the published estimates of tissue tolerances at the $TD_{5/5}$ and $TD_{50/5}$ levels for kidney, spinal cord, brain, and small intestine irradiated to one-third, two-thirds, and three-thirds of the total organ volume.

Since this data was generated by limited clinical observations of conventionally delivered radiotherapy, it serves mainly as a guideline for clinicians for conventional radiation fractionation schemes. Therefore, they do not apply directly to

Table 1.1: Normal tissue tolerance to therapeutic radiation

Organ	$TD_{5/5}$ (cGy) Organ volume			$TD_{50/5}$ (cGy) Organ volume			Objective Clinical endpoint
	1/3	2/3	3/3	1/3	2/3	3/3	
Kidney	5000	3000	2300	—	4000	2800	Nephritis
Brain	6000	5000	4500	7500	6500	6000	Necrosis
Spinal cord	5000	5000	4700	7000	7000	—	Myelitis necrosis
Small intestine	5000	—	4000	6000	—	5500	Obstruction /Perforation

Data obtained from Emani et al Int J Rad Onc Biol Phys 21(1): 109-122, 1991

the application of non-conventional regimens except in so far as the doses are translatable to equivalent biologic effects based upon the true radio-sensitivity of the organ. That is, one could assume that, using the above formula for biologic equivalent dose (BED) for the spinal cord ($\alpha/\beta = 2$), a tolerance dose of 5000cGy given in 2 Gy fractions, would yield a tolerance dose of 2867cGy if the treatment was given in 5 Gy fractions instead.

The Effect of Tissue Volume on Tissue Tolerance

As shown previously by clinical observations, it appears that radiation dose tolerances are higher if a smaller volume of a normal organ is irradiated compared to the entire organ. (See Table 1.1.) Because external beam irradiation techniques generally involve relatively large fields of radiation, clinical estimates of the tolerance of very small volumes of tissue to radiation are sparse. What is known is that tissues may vary in their radio-sensitivity, not only based on the α/β of the given tissue, but also based on the structural or functional organization of the tissue (3). The tolerance of organs may depend on their functional organization. Although the basic effect of radiation is cell killing, the tolerance of normal organs depends on the ability of clonogenic cells to maintain a sufficient number of mature cells for continued organ function. Organ function depends on the aggregation of cells into functional subunits. It has been proposed that organs can be divided into one of two types, 1) Structurally defined FSU (e.g., kidney-nephron) 2) Structurally-undefined FSU (e.g., skin, mucosa, or spinal cord) (3). In the case of the renal nephron, each nephron is a self contained structural unit independent of its neighbors. The survival of a nephron after irradiation therefore depends on at least one clonogenic cell surviving within it. Thus, the kidney may show a graded response to radiation depending on the number of surviving nephrons. Glial tissue, on the other hand, requires a sufficient number of cells per unit volume for maintenance of function. Therefore, these organs show a threshold-binary response. Others, such as intestinal crypts, behave similarly in the threshold response, but have the ability to repopulate.

Application of Radiation Principles to Radiosurgery

With the advent of new technologies in radiation therapy, re-evaluation of radiation effects must be considered. Since concepts of radiation dose tolerance were largely developed in the era of wide-field, low energy x-rays, tolerance must be revisited in the context of cellular responses, volume effects, and target tissue types.

Volume Effects

Unlike conventional irradiation which exploits the therapeutic ratio generally by fractionating a course of therapy and delivering relatively low biologic doses, radiosurgery exploits differential volume effects. While it has been previously observed that as the volume of the organ irradiated decreases, the dose to produce characteristic complications increases, volume effects in conventional irradiation have been largely ignored (6). Since the effects of increases in volume are greatest with changes in small volumes, volume effects play a more prominent role in radiosurgery as compared with conventional irradiation (3, 6). By virtue of the rapid drop-off of dose at the periphery of the target lesion, the most important radiobiologic effects are those of the target unless sensitive normal structures course through the target or the target is embedded within sensitive normal tissue. By excluding sensitive normal tissues from the high dose regions, radiosurgery allows the delivery of radiation doses large enough to transcend traditional concepts of radioresistance (7). For example, tumors such as meningiomas, schwannomas, and melanomas that are notoriously resistant to fractionated radiation regimens have a consistent favorable response to radiosurgery (7).

Dose-Volume Guidelines in Radiosurgery

Early guidelines for radiation dose prescriptions were based on iso-effect curves estimating risks of radiation necrosis from animal and clinical data (3, 9). These data confirmed that the risks of necrosis increased with increases in treated volume. Based on their initial experience using Gamma Knife radiosurgery, Flickinger et al, developed the integrated logistic predictive model of brain necrosis (9).

Tissue Tolerance to Radiosurgery

Several mathematical formulas have been proposed to equate different radiotherapy regimens. The most widely known are the exponential model and linear-quadratic models. The linear- quadratic model of radiation response is reliable for dose sizes of up to 3-5 Gy. However, the exponential model may be more reliable for single fraction radiosurgery doses (10). As an example, the estimated tolerance of the optic nerve ($\alpha/\beta = 2$), is approximately 50 Gy. If delivered as a single radiosurgical dose, the linear-quadratic model predicts a tolerance of 13.2 Gy where the exponential model predicts a dose of 9.8 Gy. Clinical observations of optic neuropathy have been seen at 9.8 Gy, suggesting that the linear-quadratic model may overestimate the tolerance of the optic nerve to radiosurgical doses (6).

The optic nerves and chiasm are known to be more sensitive than other parts of the brain to fractionated radiotherapy (10). The recommended maximum radiosurgery dose to the optic nerves is 8 Gy (11). Consequently, single fraction radiosurgery is limited in tumors of the sellar region unless the tumor is more than about 5mm from the optic nerves and chiasm. The role of fractionated stereotactic radiotherapy in this setting has been debated. With the advent of frameless radiosurgery technology such as the CyberKnife, hypofractionated regimens are possible. Clinical studies are ongoing at Stanford to define the role of hypofractionation on tumor control and risks of optic nerve injury in these patients. Additionally, the frameless technology allows the exploration of single fraction or hypofractionated treatment schedules for tumors outside of the cranium. As these uncharted areas are explored, particularly for regions where early responding tissue are included in the treated volumes, studies will need to be done to evaluate the relative effects of volume and cellular responses to unconventional radiation schedules.

References

1. Hall EJ CJ. Physical and Biologic Basis of Radiation Therapy. In: Cox JD, editor. Moss' Radiation Oncology: Rationale, Technique, Results. 7th ed. St. Louis: Mosby-Year Book, Inc.; 1994. pp. 3-66.

2. Withers HR, Thames HD. Dose fractionation and volume effects in normal tissues and tumors. Am J Clin Oncol 1988;11: 313-329.

3. Withers HR, Taylor JM, Maciejewski B. Treatment volume and tissue tolerance. Int J Radiat Oncol Biol Phys 1988;14:751-759.

4. Rubin P, Casarett, G. A Direction for Clinical Radiation Pathology. Front Radiat Ther Oncol 1972;6:1-16.

5. Emami B, Lyman J, Brown A, et al. Tolerance of normal tissue to therapeutic irradiation. Int J Radiat Oncol Biol Phys 1991;21:109-122.

6. Flickinger JC, Kondziolka D, Lunsford LD. Dose selection in stereotactic radiosurgery. Neurosurg Clin N Am 1999;10:271-280.

7. Kondziolka D, Lunsford LD, Flickinger JC. The radiobiology of radiosurgery. Neurosurg Clin N Am 1999;10:157-166.

8. Kjellberg RN, Davis KR, Lyons S, et al. Bragg peak proton beam therapy for arteriovenous malformation of the brain. Clin Neurosurg 1983;31:248-290.

9. Flickinger JC. An integrated logistic formula for prediction of complications from radiosurgery. Int J Radiat Oncol Biol Phys 1989;17:879-885.

10. Tishler RB, Loeffler JS, Lunsford LD, et al. Tolerance of cranial nerves of the cavernous sinus to radiosurgery. Int J Radiat Oncol Biol Phys 1993;27:215-221.

11. Laws ER, Jr., Vance ML. Radiosurgery for pituitary tumors and craniopharyngiomas. Neurosurg Clin N Am 1999;10:327-336.

CyberKnife Image Guidance and Tracking

Martin Murphy

Introduction

The image guidance process measures the position and orientation of the target site during treatment. In machine vision language, an object's position and orientation at a particular time are together called its pose. Pose is always defined relative to a reference position and is described by a translation matrix T involving the three translational coordinates (x,y,z) and a rotation matrix R involving the rotational angles (a,b,c) around the three coordinate axes. For CyberKnife image guidance, the patient's treatment pose is measured relative to the pose in the CT study used for treatment planning. If the pose during treatment differs from the CT pose, then T and R are applied to the beam configuration defined in the CT study to realign the beams to the new patient pose. This realignment keeps the beams, and thus the dose, in the planned geometry relative to the patient's anatomy, regardless of the patient's position during treatment.

1 Principles of Image Guidance

The pose is measured by acquiring radiographs of the patient during treatment and comparing them to corresponding digitally reconstructed radiographs (DRRs) generated from the CT treatment planning study. A complete pose determination requires two image viewpoints, for example, two fixed diagnostic x-ray cameras and two x-ray sources. The pose measurement can be based either on anatomical features or on implanted fiducials visible in the two images.

1.1 Configuration of the Imaging System

The CyberKnife uses dual diagnostic x-ray imaging systems positioned on either side of the patient couch and oriented at right angles to one another. This configuration produces a mirror-pair of oblique images in which the anterior/posterior (AP) axis of the patient runs horizontally.

The x-ray sources are approximately 3.3 meters from the detectors, to minimize interference with the robot's workspace around the patient. This distance is three times greater than for conventional diagnostic imaging and as a consequence the mAs technique used for the images is much higher than what is normally prescribed in manuals for x-ray imaging technique.

1.2 Anatomy-Based Guidance

In CyberKnife treatments all anatomy-based targeting uses bony structures in the vicinity of the target lesion. As with conventional frame-based radiosurgery, it is assumed that the target position is fixed with respect to the local skeletal landmarks. Pose estimation involves a process of image registration, in which DRRs generated from the CT study are compared to the positioning radiographs taken during treatment. Prior to treatment, a large number of possible positions of the patient are simulated and recorded in a database of precomputed DRRs; during treatment each acquired radiograph is compared to every image in the database of DRRs and a measure of similarity is computed. (The similarity measure is the cross-correlation coefficient for the pixel values in the radiograph and the comparison DRR.) The comparison process finds the best match (i.e., the largest correlation coefficient) from among the precomputed DRRs and uses that best match to determine the translation and rotation of the patient's anatomy relative to the CT.

The anatomical registration process benefits from high contrast for the bony structures. For cranial treatments the registration is determined primarily by the contour of the skull, which must be differentiated from the surface of the scalp. Imaging technique is optimized to provide the best discrimination of the skull edge.

Treatment sites at the base of the skull and top of the cervical spine are targeted using the position and orientation of the skull. Therefore, it is important to preserve the relative configuration of the skull and the articulated cervical spine vertebrae. This is accomplished with the AquaPlast mask and molded head support.

1.3 Fiducial-Based Targeting

Anatomy-based image registration of the thoracic and lumbar spine is difficult because the spine structure is complex and difficult to see in low-exposure radiographs. Soft-tissue treatment sites have no associated skeletal landmarks and are not recognizable in x-ray radiographs. To treat these sites requires the introduction of artifical landmarks called fiducials.

A fiducial is a point-like visual landmark in an object that is used to define the object's position in an image. To be useful, the fiducial must be rigidly fixed to the object so that when the object moves, the fiducial moves in exactly the same way. When this is the case, changes in the pose of the object can be inferred by observing changes in the positions of fiducials associated with the object.

A fiducial can be either a naturally-occurring point-like feature of the object, or an artificial feature attached to the object. Artificial fiducials provide clear radiographic landmarks at anatomical sites that are otherwise difficult to observe in diagnostic x-ray images. Artificial fiducials are necessary when images of the object of interest do not clearly show point-like or edge-like natural features, or when segmentation of the target object from other image structures is difficult, or when one requires greater registration accuracy than would be possible using natural anatomical features.

One or more fiducials is needed to indicate changes in the object's translational position. Three or more fiducials are needed to determine the complete pose including orientation.

If three or more fiducial landmarks on the object are visible in both camera viewpoints, then the object's pose can be represented by the coordinates $x_i = (x_i, y_i, z_i)$ of the fiducial points. These coordinates are found by back-projecting the position of each fiducial in each of the two images to its position in the object (5).

If the object changes its pose, then the fiducial coordinates change from x_i to x_i'. The change in pose is represented by a translation matrix T and a rotation matrix R. If the coordinates of all the fiducials are arranged in matrices X and X', then the change in pose is expressed mathematically as

$$X' = R\,X' + T. \qquad (1.1)$$

Fiducials allow for point-based image registration, which is the simplest, fastest, and potentially the most precise way to register images of an anatomical object in order to find the pose difference. Point-based registration is done simply by getting the fiducial coordinates x_i in the CT study, the corresponding coordinates x_i' of the same fiducials in the treatment room x-rays, and then solving equation 1.1 for the pose transformation represented by R and T.

Equation (1.1) can be solved several different ways. The most general approach involves an algebraic matrix inversion based on singular-value decomposition (7). Alternatively, the radiographic images of the fiducials can be registered to DRRs using the fiducials as the registration landmark (6). This method is a special case of the general anatomy-based registration technique. A third method finds the matrices T and R by successive approximations. It has been shown that the matrix inversion and image registration methods yield identical results (5).

1.4 The Accuracy of Image Guidance

The overall accuracy of the image guidance process depends on three separate sources of error: (1) the error in locating landmarks in the images; (2) the error in determining the pose translation and rotation from the registration process; and (3) the error in measuring the position of the diagnostic imaging system in the coordinate frame of the robot. The combined effect of these inaccuracies produces the overall target (dose) localization error, which is the precision in placing the dose at its intended location.

1.4.1 Fiducial-Based Targeting Accuracy

When the CT study and the treatment room radiographs are analyzed, there is always some uncertainty in finding the positions of the fiducials. Furthermore, in some situations it is possible for the fiducials to change their relative positions after the CT study. This results in an error (or uncertainty) in determining the pose transformation represented by R and T. If the errors (or changes) in the individual fiducial positions occur randomly, then the resulting error in the pose is reduced by increasing the number of fiducials.

The dose targeting accuracy of the CyberKnife depends on the accuracy with which the pose (position and orientation) of the treatment site is known. If the uncertainty in finding each fiducial is independent and random, then the resulting uncertainty in finding the pose of the fiducial group (and thus the target object) can be estimated. Consider a three-dimensional group of N fiducials and let σ be the uncertainty in the position of a single fiducial. The overall rms error $<dR>$ in the translation of the fiducial group is

$$<dR> = \sqrt{2\sigma^2/3N}\,\pi$$

The translational accuracy improves, but at a diminishing rate, as more fiducials are used. Using more than six fiducials offers little additional gain in accuracy (6).

The total error in the pose (combining translation and rotation) has a similar dependence on the number of fiducials, as Figure 1 shows.

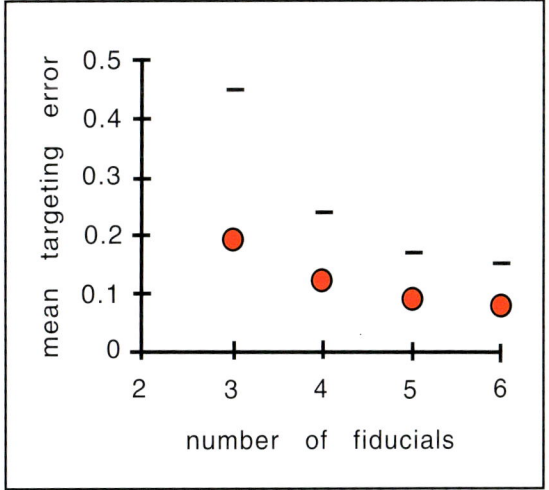

Figure 1.

The error in finding translations is unaffected by the spacing between the fiducials, provided that they do not overlap one another. The error in rotation is reduced by about half when the average distance between the fiducials is doubled.

The end-to-end targeting accuracy based on fiducials has been measured repeatedly in phantom simulation tests. After 20 such tests using a flat array of thermoluminescent detectors in a dosimetric phantom, the two-dimensional distribution of observed target centers around the intended target center looked like Figure 2, which corresponds to a 3D root-mean-square targeting error of 1.7 mm. This uncertainty combines the effects of all sources of image guidance error with the pointing accuracy of the robot and the accuracy of target localization in the treatment planning process.

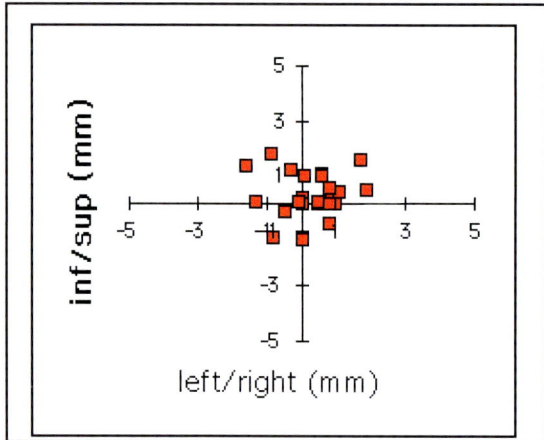

Figure 2.

1.4.2 The Accuracy of Anatomy-Based Guidance

In early tests using using a skull phantom, the average translational error for cranial registration based on anatomical landmarks was measured to be 0.3 mm along the anterior/posterior and left/right axes and 0.6 mm along the inferior/superior axis. At the same time, end-to-end dose placement tests demonstrated an overall target localization uncertainty of 1.7 mm when a CT of 1.5 mm slice spacing was used for target identification (6). In recent measurements using improved calibration, image registration, and measurement techniques, the overall dose localization uncertainty was reduced to 1.1 mm for a CT slice spacing of 1.25 mm (1). In both sets of measurements the dose placement accuracy was found to be influenced by the CT slice thickness, with more finely sliced CT images providing more accurate target definition and image registration and correspondingly smaller dose localization error.

1.5 Imaging System Calibration

The imaging system requires two independent calibrations. The first calibration establishes the intrinsic camera model for the system of two x-ray cameras. This includes the magnifications, distortions, and the relative positions and orientations of the two camera image planes. The calibration is typically performed by acquiring images of a calibration phantom consisting of a two or three-dimensional matrix of steel beads that appear as a 2D array of dots on the image planes. By imaging a single calibration phantom simultaneously with both cameras, it is possible to calibrate the imaging system as a unit. This calibration typically does not change unless the cameras and/or sources are physically moved.

The second calibration establishes the spatial position of the camera coordinate system with respect to the robot coordinate system. This calibration is a critical element in the targeting accuracy of the CyberKnife because any residual error is systematic and causes a fixed offset of the dose distribution from its intended location. This calibration can typically be determined to within +/- 0.5 mm along each coordinate axis. This relative position of the two coordinate systems is represented by a fixed offset vector (x,y,z) that is nonzero except in the unlikely case that the robot's virtual isocenter exactly coincides with the camera coordinate origin. The offset vector typically changes only if the camera system is moved or the robot is remastered. It is of critical importance to perform periodic QA tests to verify that this offset has not changed. This can be accomplished by making several consecutive end-to-end tests that record absolute targeting error. If the mean dose (target) localization error systematically differs from zero by more than 0.5 mm, then it is likely that the robot/camera offset has changed and should be recalibrated.

2 Clinical Operations Relevant to Image Guidance

2.1 The Use of Fiducials during Treatment

In CyberKnife spine radiosurgery, the treatment site is rigidly associated with the spine, which itself is made up of connected rigid bodies (the vertebral segments). Metal fiducials attached to a single vertebral body show clearly in x-rays of the thoracic and lumbar spine, allowing rapid point-based registration of treatment targets that are otherwise difficult to detect in the treatment room images.

For lung radiosurgery, the target tumor itself cannot be effectively discerned and it is not rigidly associated with any natural radiographic landmarks. Fiducials implanted in the tumor itself provide artificial point landmarks for image registration. Unlike fiducials imbedded in the spine, soft-tissue fiducials can move relative to one another, resulting in an additional source of uncertainty in measuring the pose of the treatment target.

A minimum of three fiducials should be used. Accuracy improves when more than three fiducials are used, but the improvement diminishes with each additional fiducial. The fiducials should be arranged 2 - 3 cm apart and such that there is a clear line of sight for each fiducial along the oblique viewpoint of the imaging system. This requires some visual estimation by the clinician implanting the fiducials. If the patient has other radio-opaque materials that will show up in the treatment room radiographs (e.g., surgical clips, spine orthopedic hardware, dense calcium deposits in the bone, etc.) the fiducials should be placed so that they will not be obstructed by the other materials along the lines of sight of the x-ray cameras.

If more than three fiducials are in place, then any three (or more) will provide a complete measurement of the patient pose. This allows some redundancy for situations where a fiducial moves or turns out to be hard to see. Migration of the fiducials within the anatomy can be detected by comparing their relative spacing in the CT study with their spacing during treatment. Because it is unlikely that fiducials will migrate as a fixed cluster, stability in their spacing can be interpreted as stability in their anatomical position.

Generally, the fiducials should be at least 2 mm in their largest dimension. i.e., if the fiducials are spheres, they should have a diameter • 2 mm; if the fiducials are elongated, then they should be • 2 mm along their longest axis.

Spine fiducials should be steel, gold, or tantalum pins or screws that can be firmly attached to bone. Aluminum, titanium, plastic, or other low-Z fiducials do not provide sufficient contrast against bone.

Soft-tissue fiducials can be steel or gold seeds, surgical clips, or balls. When possible, the fiducials should be anchored to tissue with sutures. Four to six fiducials should be placed around the perimeter of the tumor, at least 2 - 3 cm apart, avoiding overlap along the lines of sight for the imaging system.

At the time of CT imaging, one should also acquire radiographic images of the patient with the CyberKnife system. This will verify that at least three, and preferably all fiducials are visible, clearly separated, and not overlapped by other radio-opaque objects.

Any fiducial shifting or migration that occurs between the day of the CT study and the treatment day will degrade the accuracy of fiducial-based targeting. In extreme cases, it can render the case untreatable. During the 24 hour period immediately following implantation, the fiducial positions can potentially be affected by swelling and other transient reactions to the procedure. Subsequent fiducial movement is likely to progress more slowly over time. Therefore, it is recommended to wait at least 24 hours following implantation before acquiring the treatment planning CT study, and then to minimize the time between CT study and treatment.

2.2 Imaging Frequency

The clinician has considerable discretion in setting the frequency of imaging during treatment. More imaging will improve the accuracy of dose placement but will prolong the duration of treatment. Therefore, setting the frequency requires a tradeoff between treatment accuracy and efficiency.

Five years of treatment records at Stanford have provided a basis for estimating the effects of imaging frequency on the accuracy of dose placement. These records, which show the character and frequency of movement for several hundred skull and spine patients, have recently been published (3). Based on statistical inference it can be concluded that for the average patient, an imaging interval of 1 - 2 minutes is sufficient to keep more than 98% of the dose within 2 mm of the planned position. However, there is considerable variation among patients, with a small percentage showing more than the usual amount and magnitude of movement. Therefore, for each patient the real-time position record should be monitored for evidence of too much movement and the clinician should be prepared to modify the imaging regimen during the fraction(s) as needed.

References

1. Chang SD, Main W, Martin DP, et al, An analysis of the accuracy of the CyberKnife: a robotic frameless stereotactic radiosurgical system, Neurosurgery 52:140 - 147, 2003

2. Murphy MJ: The importance of computed tomography slice thickness in radiographic patient positioning for radiosurgery. Med Phys 26:171-175, 1999

3. Murphy MJ, Chang SD, Gibbs IC: Patterns of patient movement during frameless image-guided radiosurgery. Int J Rad Onc Biol Phys 55:1400-1408, 2003

4. Murphy MJ, Martin D, Whyte R: The effectiveness of breath-holding to stabilize lung and pancreas tumors during radiosurgery. Int J Rad Onc Biol Phys 53:475-482, 2002

5. Murphy MJ: Fiducial-based targeting accuracy for external-beam radiotherapy. Med Phys 29: 334 - 344, 2002

6. Murphy MJ and Cox RS: The accuracy of dose localization for an image-guided frameless radiosurgery system. Medical Physics 23: 2043 - 2049, 1996

7. Schonemann P: A generalized solution of the orthogonal procrustes problem. Psychometrika 31: 1 - 10 (1966).

CyberKnife Physics and Quality Assurance

Anthony Ho

Introduction

The CyberKnife linac operates in the X band (9300 MHz), which makes it smaller and lighter than a conventional S band (2856 MHz) medical linac. The X band linac is supposed to give a lower output than the S band units. In fact, the original prototype unit at Stanford only gave an output of 300 cGy per minute at 80 cm. But the new generation CyberKnife is capable of providing an output of over 400 MU/min. However, users of the system should be aware that the dose linearity will worsen when dose rate is increased from 300 to 400 MU/min. In addition, the calibration of the machine will change when the dose rate is changed. It is extremely important to check the output, e.g., after the service engineer adjusts the magnetron parameters such as the magnetron current or the pulse repetition frequency, because the output of the unit will change.

The robot provides the automated positioning and pointing of the beam at the target. There are limitations on how many solid angles are available because the robotic arm must not come in contact with the patient, the table, or the imaging system, and it must not point the treatment beam directly into the imaging system. We conduct monthly checks for the whole delivery system using two different phantoms. Additionally, the imaging system is checked by Accuray engineers during routine preventive maintenance inspection. If the monthly check using Thermoluminescent Dosimeters (TLD) or film indicates that the whole system is functioning correctly, it is not necessary to individually check the robot or the imaging system on a monthly basis. We use TLD for our routine QA tests, but we also used films during commissioning and for other testing of the system.

During commissioning of the system, the equipment is tested extensively. For routine clinical use, quality assurance is performed to verify that the CyberKnife system is acceptable for clinical use. The following is a brief summary of the quality assurance being done at Stanford.

Morning Calibration Check

A Farmer chamber fixed to the jig is used everyday when there are patients to be treated. Once a day measurement is sufficient since the room temperature is very stable and the atmospheric pressure does not change too much during the day. We have measured the output many times both in the morning and afternoon, and the variations were very minimal. Figure 1 shows the form that we use at Stanford for the morning calibration. There are items which are checked but do not appear on the form. We also write down the MU/min., and check the chiller temperature, which should be constant at 18 degree C for our unit. *The machine calibration factor is entered in the CyberKnife system for both the primary and secondary dosimeters.*

Monthly Calibration QA

A different Farmer chamber with solid water is being used every month to cross check the Farmer chamber used with the jig. Figure 2 is the form used for the monthly QA, while Figure 3 shows some comparison of the two Farmer chambers. The energy is also checked by taking the ionization readings at two different depths and taking the ratio of the two readings. Central axis laser alignment and symmetry of the beam are also checked with film, and the symmetry result is analyzed by the RIT film scanner. A typical result is shown in Figure 4. In addition, the safety interlocks are checked, and the in-room radiation detectors are also checked.

Monthly TLD Check – Fiducial Tracking

Fiducials are being used in a Solid Water phantom to perform the monthly check, alternating months using the horizontal and vertical setups. Approximately 47 TLDs are used for each setup. The Harshaw TLD microchips (1x1x1 mm) are used with a Harshaw automatic TLD reader (model 5500). A 15 mm diameter collimator is used for the horizontal setup and a 25 mm diameter collimator is used for the vertical setup. Since the TLDs are located on a single slab, therefore, only two profiles can be checked at a time. Figure 5 shows comparison of the dose profile from TLD and from the treatment planning system. The CIRS head phantom as described in the following section may also be used for the monthly check if fiducials are put in the insert of the phantom. The Solid Water phantom is scanned using 1.5 mm CT slices. For TLD calibration, 100 MU is used with a SSD of 78.5 cm at a depth of 1.5 cm using a 60 mm collimator. The TLD supralinearity is being corrected. Using more TLDs allows us to accurately determine the shift of the centroid when comparing the dose profile from the planning system with the dose determined from the TLD.

Monthly TLD Check – Skull Tracking

The CIRS head phantom is used for the monthly check of the skull tracking accuracy. The custom made TLD cube has the dimension of 6.35 x 6.35 x 6.35 cm, with 2-mm thick tissue equivalent slabs. The central plate has 61 holes, diameter 1.5 mm, depth 1 mm, to accommodate the same microchips used for the fiducials tracking test. The spacing of the TLD holes in the cassette is 2-mm center to center. Other plates have a single hole in the center. A 0.625 mm CT slice thickness is used and fewer TLDs are used for the skull tracking test. Seven TLDs are used and they are arranged in three dimensions so that accuracy along right-left, anterior-posterior, and superior-inferior directions is checked at the same time. The 5 mm collimator is used and by using the small diameter collimator with a single isocenter plan, it is possible to ascertain spatial accuracy of treatment delivery using a small number of TLDs. The measurements are repeated two more times, and the average of the three groups of TLD readings are used to verify that the beams are aiming at the center of the TLD array, as shown in Figure 6. A dose of 800 cGy is delivered to the 90% isodose line. For TLD calibration, 800 cGy is delivered with the same phantom setup as used in the fiducials tracking test. Results show that the beam is delivered to within 1 mm of the TLD array center. Repeated measurements show similar results indicating that the CyberKnife, as well as the TLD system, are both stable and consistent.

Treatment Planning System QA

The fiducial tracking monthly QA plan is recalculated every few months, and the skull tracking monthly QA plan is calculated every month. The TLD test results also serve the purpose of checking the CyberKnife treatment planning system. A good quality assurance procedure should also include a Physics second check of the monitor unit (MU) calculation output from the treatment planning system. The CyberKnife typically utilizes approximately 100 to 150 beams to deliver a treatment. For the Physics check of the monitor unit, we have been picking one of the beams and confirming the monitor unit with hand calculation. In order to check all the beams, a simple program has been developed to facilitate the calculation. The program reads the CyberKnife output file, which includes the information on the collimator size, source to calculation point distance, the effective depth, the off axis distance, the dose to that point, as well as the monitor unit to deliver that dose. The program is being run in a shell tool or command window on any PC. The calculation is carried out for each beam and summed for the total dose: Dose = OF x TPR x OAR x $1/R^2$ x MU where OF is the output factor, TPR is the tissue phantom ratio, OAR is the off axis ratio, and $1/R^2$ is the inverse square correction. The program compares the CyberKnife TPS dose calculation and the secondary check result. Figure 7 shows the single point MU calculation and Figure 8 gives an example of the MU calculation program, which calculates all the beams.

Whole System QA

The treatment plans for both the monthly TLD checks (fiducials tracking and skull tracking) are re-calculated often. Therefore the whole system, including the treatment planning system, the robot system, the imaging system, as well as the treatment process, is tested when the monthly TLD readings indicate consistent and accurate results.

Treatment Plan Evaluation (Physics)

Figure 9 shows a form called Treatment Plan Evaluation (Physics). We routinely have a second Physics check, which includes evaluating the treatment plan, etc. As part of the QA, record keeping is also important. Therefore keeping a database of all the patients treated should be part of the complete QA process. We use an Excel spreadsheet to keep a small database of all the patients being treated.

QA during Treatment

During treatment, it is important that the CyberKnife team members observe the treatment console and the video monitor closely. This is important especially for the fiducial tracking treatments because the software program sometimes picks up noise near the real fiducials and gives a false robot correction reading. In such case, the operator either re-takes the image or finds out what else can be done to correct such false reading. The central laser is left on during treatments just to have a visual check of where the beam is aiming.

Miscellaneous

The room lasers are not checked routinely because their accuracy is not too important. The lasers are left on during the week and the drifting is minimal. An annual or biannual calibration of the unit should be performed. The proper operation of the video monitors and intercom system should be part of the daily QA process. Unusual noise and smell which come from the machine should be investigated, and routine visual inspection of the unit should be part of a good QA program.

Figure 1

PRETREATMENT CALIBRATION

Warming up: _____ MU. **SF$_6$ pressure:** _____

Room Temperature: _____ ºC; **Pressure :** _____ mmHg
(Parameter placed on the couch).

$$C_{T,P} = \frac{273+t}{295} * \frac{760}{p} =$$

Setup: Attach the Pretreatment Calibration Jig to the Cyberknife, with the 60 mm collimator in place.

    Electrometer (K602, s/n 31617A): Bias: -300V; Scale: $10*10^{-8}$C; Display: 10V.
    Set CyberKnife calibration factors to 1.00. Deliver 200 MU.

Reading: ($*10^{-8}$C) _____ **R$_{ave}$:** _____

    Calibration Factor = 1 / (R$_{ave}$ *C$_{T,P}$ *0.224) =
Enter Calibration Factor (use same factor for channels A and B) in N1000 software.
Repeat measurement, making sure output is within 1.0% of 1.00 cGy/MU.

Reading: ($*10^{-8}$C) _____ **R$_{ave}$:** _____

Physicist: _____ ; Date: _____

Figure 2

CyberKnife Monthly Calibration

Date: _____ ; Physicist: _____ ; SF$_6$ pressure: _____

Chamber: _____

Electrometer : _____

Room Temperature: _____ °C; Pressure : _____

$$C_{T,P} = \frac{273+t}{295} * \frac{760}{p} =$$

1. **Setup for Dose rate**: Solid water phantom, 78.5cm SSD, depth=3.0 cm, Coll= 60 mm. Set CyberKnife calibration factors to 1.00. Deliver 200 MU.
    Reading: (*10^{-8}C) _____ ; **R$_{ave}$**: _____
    Dose rate = R$_{ave}$ _____ * C$_{T,P}$ _____ *0.268 = _____ (Rad/MU)
    Expected dose rate to water: <u>1.006</u> (Calibration data on 11/7/2001)

2. **Check for CyberKnife Calibration Factors**:
    Calibration Factor = 1/(R$_{ave}$ *C$_{T,P}$ *0.268)=
    Enter Calibration Factor (use same factor for channel A and B)
    Repeat measurements, making sure output is within 1.0% of 1.00 cGy/MU.
    Reading: (*10^{-8}C) _____ **R$_{ave}$**: _____
    % Deviation = R$_{ave}$ *C$_{T,P}$ _____ / 3.732 = _____

3. **Energy Check**:
    Add two pieces of polystyrene phantom on top (~ 5.25 cm).
    Reading: (*10^{-8}C) _____ **R$_{ave}$**: _____
    Ratio: _____ ; Expected: <u>0.811</u>;

4. **Central Axis Laser Alignment Check**:
    XV film at depth = 3.0 cm solid water phantom. Turn on the laser and mark the point with a push pin on the film. 78.5cm SSD, Collimator = 60 mm and MU= 40.

5. **Flatness and symmetry check**:
    XV film at depth=5.0 cm solid water phantom. SSD=78.5cm, Coll=40 mm and MU=40.

6. **Safety and interlock check**:
    Door: _____; E_Stop: _____; Radiation Indicator: _____.

Figure 3

Chamber Intercomparison

Date	PTW Reading	Accuray jig reading	Ratio: Accuray/PTW
12-5-2001	3.750 x 0.986	4.441 x 0.983	1.181
1-3-2002	3.751 x 0.984	4.4927 x 0.984	1.198
2-4-2002	3.742 x 0.985	4.4212 x 0.985	1.182
3-5-2002	3.740 x 0.992	4.448 x 0.992	1.189
4-8-2002	3.713 x 0.992	4.409 x 0.992	1.187
5-3-2002	3.708 x 0.992	4.370 x 0.992	1.179
6-10-2002	3.704 x 1.004	4.398 x 1.004	1.187
7-1-2002	3.731 x 0.9984	4.416 x 0.9961	1.181
8-2-2002	3.724 x 0.9994	4.415 x 0.9994	1.186
9-3-2002	3.584 x 0.9974	4.262 x 0.9974	1.189
10-18-2002	3.623 x 0.9975	4.315 x 0.9935	1.186
11-5-2002	3.650 x 0.9877	4.396 x 0.9877	1.204
12-3-2002	3.708 x 0.9870	4.413 x 0.9870	1.190
1-2-2003	3.664 x 0.9838	4.370 x 0.9838	1.193
2-7-2003	3.646 x 0.9922	4.340 x 0.9909	1.189

Figure 4

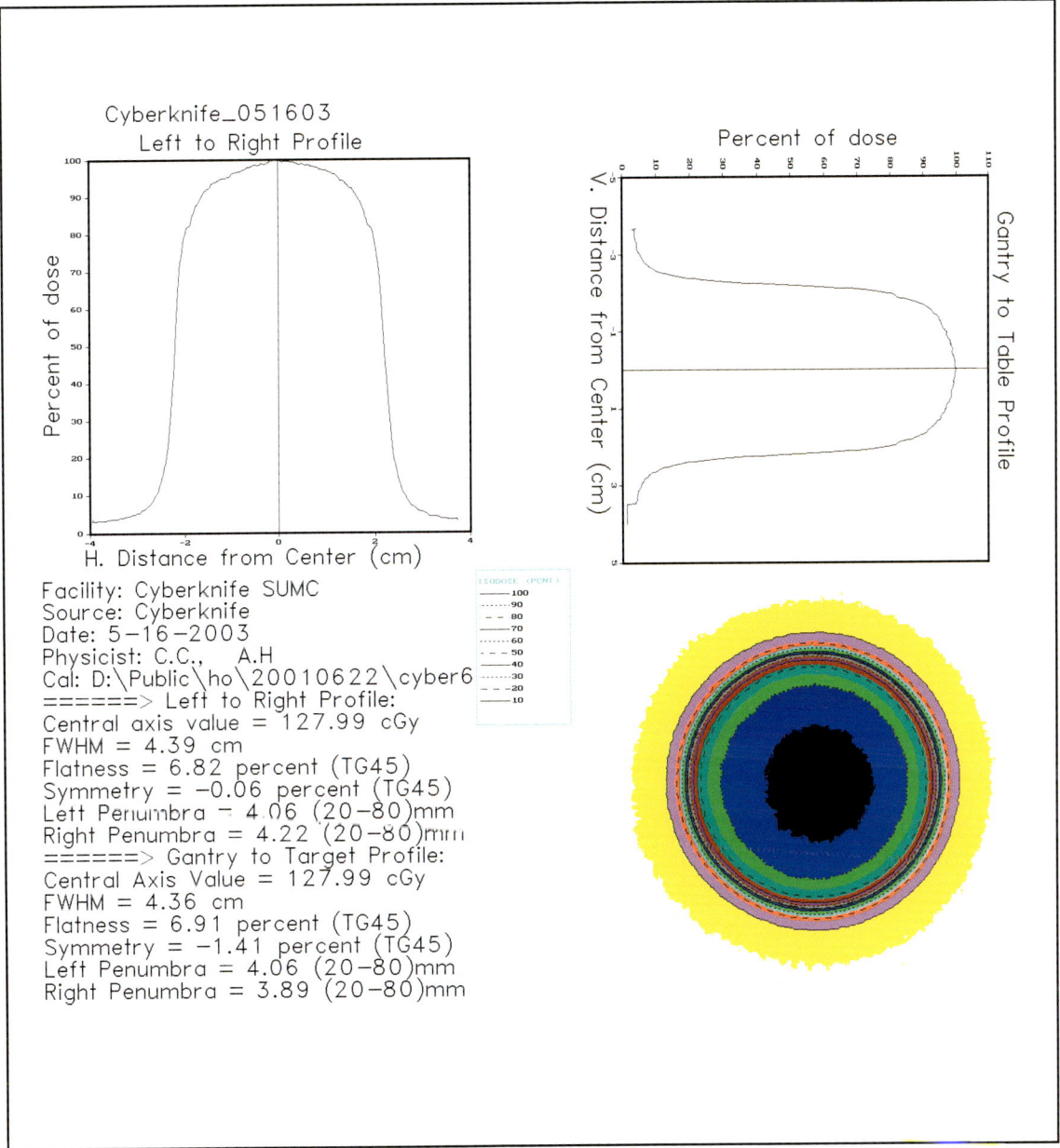

Figure 5

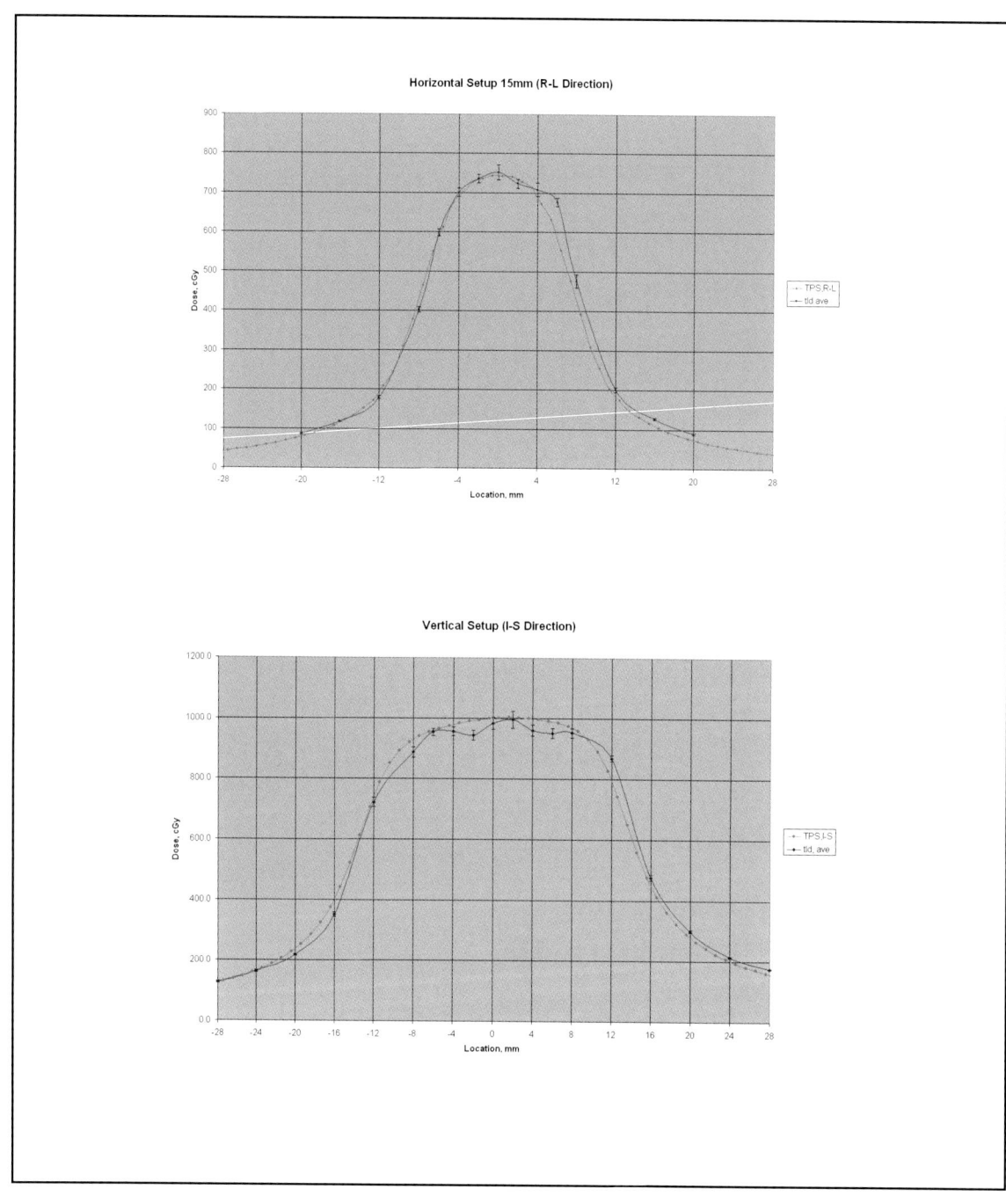

Figure 6

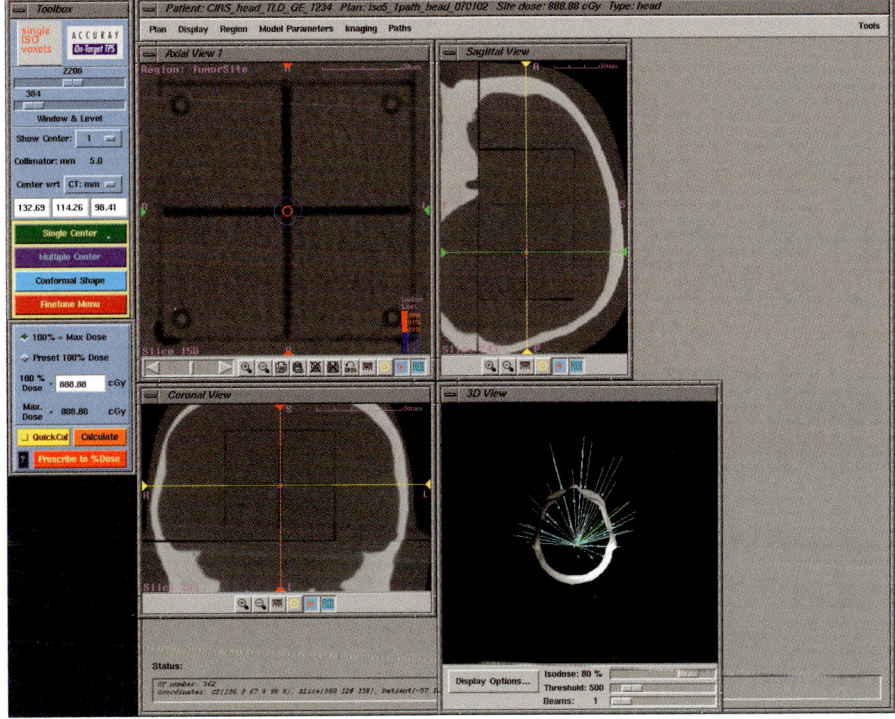

Figure 7

Patient Name   _____

MU HAND CALCULATION

$$MU = \frac{Dose\ per\ Fraction\ (cGy)}{\left(1\ ^{cGy}/_{MU}\right)\left(80.0cm/SAD(cm)\right)^2 (TPR(Depth, Field\ Size))\left(^{NPSF(Actual\ Field\ Size)}/_{NPSF(Coll\ Field\ Size)}\right)(OF(Coll\ Field\ Size))}$$

Calc. Check   Path: $MU_{TPS} =$

                    Node: $MU_{Calc} =$

Calc. done by _____

DOUBLE CHECK

Treatment plan on treatment sheet is available for patient named on treatment sheet   ____

The plan prescription (dose and fractionation) agrees with the Radiation Oncologist's signed prescription   ____

Plan has been reviewed   ____

Check done by _____

Figure 8

Example of a typical printout of the MU calculation program:

```
CyberKnife Dose Calculation Program
Version Number Version 1.0, FEBRUARY 2003AD
System Time:
9:48:51  3 / 1 / 2003
Printing a selection of Beams
Beam    27      3/1    7.5 102.6    6.4 mu 148.70 DOSE :=    5.92
     OPf  0.8090 TMRf  0.6412 ISQf  0.9133 OARf  0.0840 cGy Per MU :=
 0.0398
Beam    48      4/1    7.5 107.9    5.4 mu 151.14 DOSE :=   13.13
     OPf  0.8090 TMRf  0.6254 ISQf  0.9243 OARf  0.1858 cGy Per MU :=
 0.0869
Beam   155     13/1    7.5 118.5    9.3 mu 151.14 DOSE :=    1.13
     OPf  0.8090 TMRf  0.5930 ISQf  0.9008 OARf  0.0173 cGy Per MU :=
 0.0075
Beam   248     21/1    7.5 132.4    5.1 mu 151.14 DOSE :=   13.55
     OPf  0.8090 TMRf  0.5514 ISQf  0.8587 OARf  0.2340 cGy Per MU :=
 0.0896
Beam   345     29/1    7.5  84.4    5.2 mu 151.14 DOSE :-   16.54
     OPf  0.8090 TMRf  0.7050 ISQf  0.8864 OARf  0.2164 cGy Per MU :=
 0.1094
Beam   370     31/1    7.5 110.2    3.1 mu 151.14 DOSE :=   50.65
     OPf  0.8090 TMRf  0.6194 ISQf  0.9695 OARf  0.6898 cGy Per MU :=
 0.3351
Beam   405     34/1    7.5  56.5    4.5 mu 151.14 DOSE :=   37.51
```
  Successfully Completed Calculation

Figure 9

CyberKnife Treatment Plan Evaluation (Physics)

Patient Name: _____

Plan Name: _____ Date:_____

<u>Tumor and Dose Matrix Statistics:</u> Stages: _____

Reference Dose _____ Gy at _____ % Single Isocenter (y/n)? _____

Maximum Dose _____Gy at _____% Dose to Reference _____cGy

Total Tumor Volume: _____ cm^3; PIV/TIV: _____; TIV*PIV/(TV)^2: _____

Max. transverse_____cm; Perp. transverse_____cm; Vertical_____cm;

Coverage isodose line (total tumor volume being covered)_____% _____Gy/__stg

Tumor volume treated at ref. dose: _____ cm^3, _____% of total volume ____Gy/__stg

Tumor volume treated at 80% ref. dose: _____cm^3, _____% of total volume ___Gy/__stg

Tumor volume treated at 50% ref. dose: _____cm^3, _____% of total volume ___Gy/__stg

Total volume of non-target tissue treated at 100% reference dose _____cm^3 _____Gy/__stg

Total volume of non-target tissue treated at coverage isodose _____cm^3 _____Gy/__stg

Total volume of non-target tissue treated at 80% reference dose _____cm^3 _____Gy/__stg

Total volume of non-target tissue treated at 50% reference dose _____cm^3 _____Gy/__stg

<u>Critical Structures:</u>

Total Volume of the structure:

Total volume treated at 100% reference dose _____cm^3 _____Gy/__stg

Total volume treated at coverage isodose _____cm^3 _____Gy/__stg

Total volume treated at 80% reference dose _____cm^3 _____Gy/__stg

Total volume treated at 50% reference dose _____cm^3 _____Gy/__stg

Total volume treated at 20% reference dose _____cm^3 _____Gy/__stg

Planned By: _____

Checked by:_____; Date: _____

The Treatment Planning System

M. Peter Heilbrun
Derek Olender

Introduction

The CyberKnife robotic manipulator can aim the beams emanating from the miniature linac at potentially thousands of points within a target volume. Unlike isocentric radiation delivery systems, this capability greatly expands the number of potential solutions for generating highly homogeneous and conformal dose distributions. Such solutions have a steep dose gradient which is important in limiting radiation damage to tissues adjacent to the target volume. These non-isocentric delivery plans are generated by an inverse solution iterative process. That is, the operator assigns minimum dose values to target volume borders and maximum dose values to surrounding adjacent critical structures, and the plan selects the optimal set of beams to fit those parameters. Additionally, plans generated as an inverse solution can be individually fine tuned by adding and removing specific beams and changing beam doses. For example, eliminating or adjusting the dose of some beams that pass through critical structures or structures containing air can improve a computer generated inverse solution. This chapter will describe the methods used by the Stanford radiosurgery team to extend and optimize some of the routines presented in the Accuray On-Target Treatment Planning System Clinical User's Guide.

1. Treatment Planning Modules and Path Selection

The CyberKnife team has developed treatment planning software modules that efficiently coordinate the system's complex components to generate different treatment plans for different parts of the body. For example, the radiosurgery team does not have to start from scratch from the potentially infinite number of beam trajectories surrounding a target volume. Instead, after loading the appropriate imaging studies, the operator is prompted to choose among sets of predetermined beam trajectories termed paths. These paths are a set number of approximately 110 robot manipulator positions or vectors from which the linac beams can be fired. At each beam position there is an additional set of 12 different directions or vectors from which to aim the beam. This combination of over 1320 vectors or beam positions within a 3D space is termed the solid angle within which the beam positions reside. The beam positions in each path are pre-selected to provide the largest possible solid angle from which to deliver beams to a target volume. These paths also eliminate beam positions that could be directed at the image cameras, and robot positions that could result in linac or robot collision with the patient table and cameras.

The non-isocentric capability of the CyberKnife results from the combination of up to 12 beam vectors at each of the 110 linac positions. It is this combination which allows the beams to be aimed at any point within a target volume. In actual practice, optimal target volume conformality is achieved when beams are aimed at points that conform to the three dimensional border or boundary of the target volume. The operator can adjust these points to specific distances both inside and outside the target volume border.

Once the paths are selected, the operator can select classic modes of beam delivery, such as single and multiple isocenter techniques, which may be sufficient for target volumes that are nearly spherical and not contiguous to critical structures. However, in light of the CyberKnife's unique capability for treating non-spherical asymmetric target volumes and for maximally protecting adjacent structures, in most cases, the operator would choose to use the conformal technique. Selection of one or more of these menus starts the operator along a practical course for generating an acceptable treatment plan, *i.e.*, a plan that produces a maximal, relatively homogeneous and conformal dose of radiation to the target volume through a configuration of beam trajectories and dose weighting, and that simultaneously minimizes the dose to the operator defined adjacent critical structures.

2. Conformal Inverse Planning

Most linac and cobalt-60 radiosurgery systems use forward planning, by which the operator manually selects specific arcs or helmet aperture blocks and then evaluates the dose distribution using those beam positions. Minor adjustments can be made if the dose distribution through the target volumes and adjacent critical structures is not satisfactory. By contrast, conformal CyberKnife plans use inverse planning algorithms. At its most basic level, inverse planning simply requires the operator to assign a minimal dose to a target volume border in order to attain a highly conformal and homogeneous dose to the target volume with an acceptable dose gradient. However, to attain acceptable dose gradients when critical anatomic structures are adjacent to the target volume, the operator may need to assign maximal doses to those critical structures. Additionally, the operator can construct an array of artificial barriers or dose constraint structures which also serve to limit dose to anatomic structures. The inverse planning algorithms then attempt to generate a solution, i.e., to select a combination of beams that best fit the dose criteria. The algorithms deal with the constraining structures first. Once the constraint criteria are met, the algorithms then select the beams that generate the best conformal target volume dose.

In the absence of any adjacent critical structures, inverse planning can generally derive an acceptable selection of beams that provides a conformal dose. However, in the presence of critical structures, a solution or acceptable plan may be more difficult to attain; in some cases, the critical structures may so constrain the computation that no acceptable plan can be generated. Thus, to generate solutions in the conformal planning mode, after defining the target volume, one must concentrate on the critical, constraining structures. Examples are the optic nerves, the chiasm and the globes adjacent to peri-optic lesions, the brain stem adjacent to vestibular schwannomas, and the spinal cord adjacent to vertebral lesions.

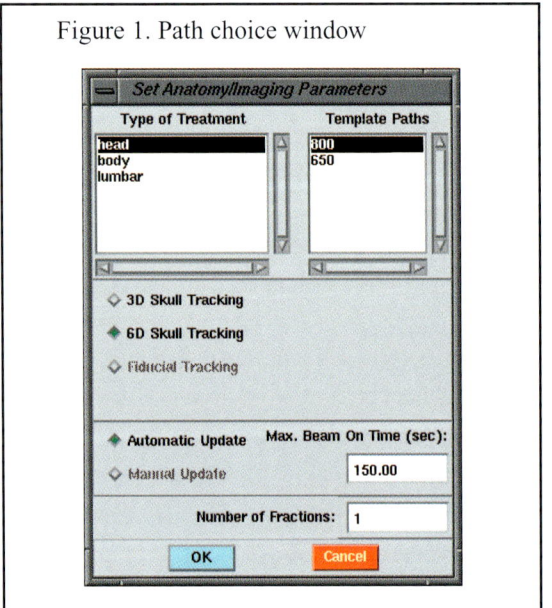

Figure 1. Path choice window

The easiest way to position a constraint is to outline the anatomic critical structure. However, if the constraint is a large structure such as the brain stem, outlining the whole structure may result in prolonging the computation process if the dose to every voxel in that specific constraint volume is assessed in the computation. Several methods are available to position artifical barriers or constraints in such cases. For example, the operator can draw in separate points, lines, open and closed curves, and small volumes which act to block beams. Learning how to select and use these various types of constraints is essential to generating acceptable CyberKnife conformal plans. Keeping the concept of constraints in mind makes the process of designing acceptable treatment plans practical, intuitive, and understandable.

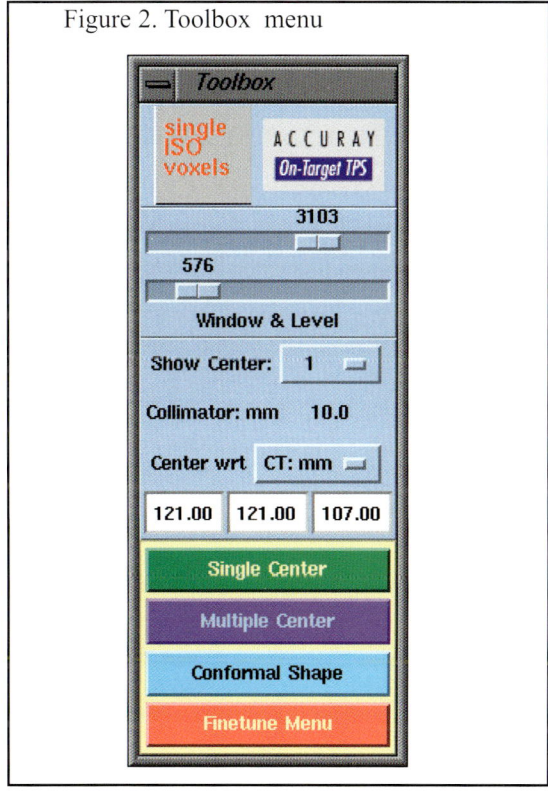

Figure 2. Toolbox menu

3. Checklists to Generate a Treatment Plan

The following checklists represent the basic steps for treatment planning.

A. Delineation of Regions of Interest, Target Volume, and Critical Structures

1) Load the CT or CT/MR fused images and review them displayed in the axial, sagittal and coronal views.

2) Decide which are the regions of interest and identify their borders. (These regions of interest are generally the target structures to be ablated and the anatomic critical structures that need to be protected.)

3) Identify the lesions or target volumes and outline them using the system drawing tools.

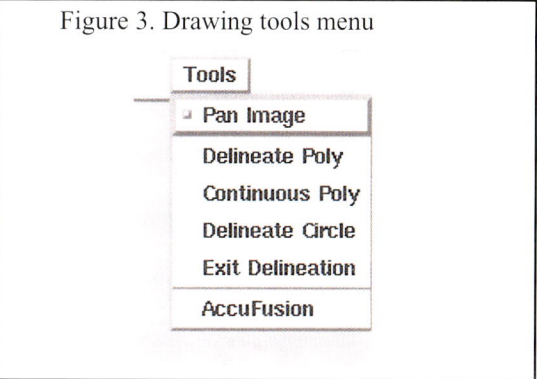

Figure 3. Drawing tools menu

4) Determine the proximity of the lesions or target volumes to the normal anatomic structures and decide if those structures, whether of normal or distorted shape, or of normal or compromised function, are critical structures for constraining the planning solution.

B. Outlining Target Volumes

After the operator has surveyed and catalogued the target volumes and critical structures in a case:

1) Open the DISPLAY pull-down menu to see if the default list includes the names of the identified structures. If not, add the name(s). (All of the structure names and general categories such as critical can be edited and customized by the operator.)

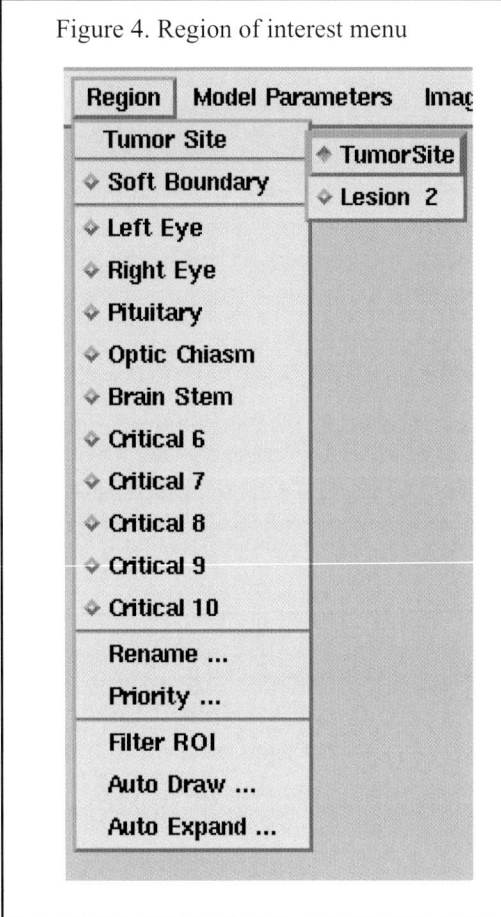

Figure 4. Region of interest menu

2) Initiate the manual outlining of the selected regions of interest with the point and click feature of the screen cursor.

It is reasonable to start with definition of the target volume by bringing up a top, bottom, or central scan slice. This area should then be magnified. It should be noted that every point placed or deposited along a structure border is entered into the plan computation. Thus, placing the fewest points that satisfactorily define the structure border is more efficient than using the continuous point deposition. The operator then outlines the target volume borders in each of the axial scan slices in which the structure is visualized. As the target volume builds slice by slice, its colored outline can also be viewed simultaneously in the sagittal, coronal, and 3D volume windows. It is important to visualize the outline in each of the three standard windows to monitor how the volume being drawn in the axial window builds in the other views. This visualization in all three views may alert the operator to discrepancies in drawn target borders from slice to slice. Adjustments can be made by deleting points with the right mouse button and re-depositing points with the left mouse button. See Figure 5.

3) Save and label the plan.

As each of the target volumes is outlined, it is good practice to save the plan, labeling it with an understandable name like "anatomy." After a single target volume outline is completed and saved, one goes through the same process with additional target volumes. Individual structures being outlined must be highlighted in the pull down DISPLAY menu and their labels should be noted in the top of the axial window. The points being outlined will appear brighter in the window than the points of structures already outlined.

C. Management of Critical or Constraint Structures

As with the target volume, the treatment plan computation uses all of the deposited points and their enclosed volumes. Therefore, when defining critical or constraint structures, one should consider methods to reduce the number of deposited points. The most rational method is to outline the borders of the critical structure by the same point deposition method used in defining a target volume. However, in some cases, this may result in an impractically large number of points, which could increase the treatment plan computation time, possibly to hours. Although this might be necessary for critical structures such as the optic nerves, the optic chiasm, and the brain stem or spinal cord, the other methods of building artifical constraints may be effective to mark critical structures without unduly increasing computation time. Each operator should decide on a case by case basis the most suitable constraint methods. Several examples of these methods can be considered as follows:

Before deciding to use constraints, it is useful to generate a plan using only appropriately sized collimators and no constraints. For example, in the case of a vestibular schwanomma shown in Figure 5, using a 12.5 mm collimator and assigning a minimal dose to the target volume border of 1800 cGy and a maximal dose of 2200 cGy to the whole target volume generated a plan with a dose distribution that is highly conformal to the target volume border at the 1800 cGy (80%) isodose. The dose is relatively homogeneous within the 1800 to 2200 cGy range. However, in this solution, the selected beams also extend the 1100 cGy (50%) isodose into the posterior brain stem. At this point the operator must consider which constraint method would best compress the 50% isodose line towards the target volume border without compromising the conformality and homogeneity to the target volume.

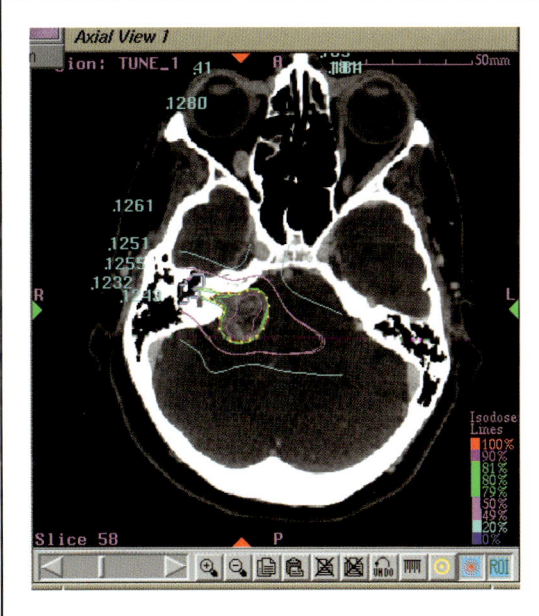

Figure 5. No constraints
Note extension of 50% magenta isodose curve into the brain stem.

Method 1. Outline the boundary or surface of the critical structure that is adjacent to the target volume.

In Figure 6, the operator has outlined the brain stem which has been assigned a maximal dose of 1700 cGy. The generated plan shows only a minimal reduction in the 50 % dose to the brain stem. However, when a maximal dose lower than 1700 cGy was assigned to the brain stem, the algorithm could not find a solution. The difficulty results from using the whole volume of the brain stem as a constraint. Since only the portion of the brain stem which is adjacent to the target volume requires dose reduction, it is more efficient to establish a constraint by drawing a barrier which serves as a wall or a shell between the target volume and the critical anatomic structure. These alternatives are described in Methods 2 and 3.

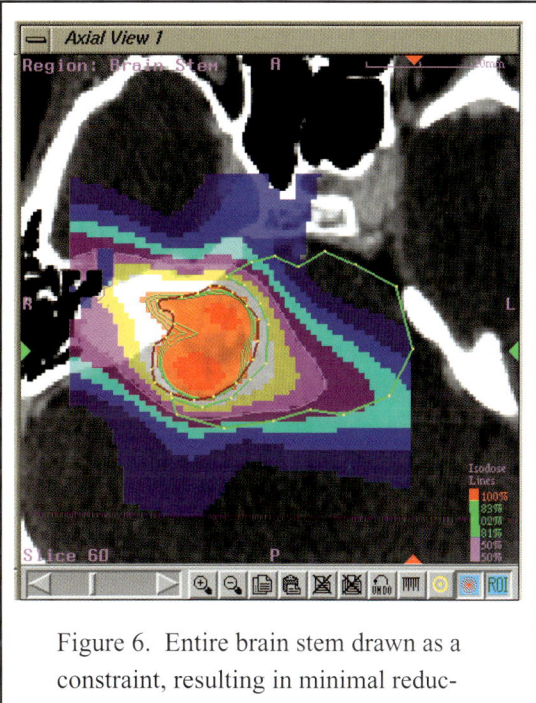

Figure 6. Entire brain stem drawn as a constraint, resulting in minimal reduction of 50% isodose.

Method 2. Deposit constraints which can be

a) a point or a line either within or outside a target volume,

b) an open curve either within or outside a target volume, or

c) a closed curve either within or outside of a target volume.

This function (Method 2) is accessed through the INVERSE PLANNING dialog window by opening the button labeled Set Manual in the Constraint Selection box.

Figure 7 shows several points that are deposited and connected to form an open curve around the anterior, inferor, and medial margin of the target volume with an assigned maximal dose of 1700 cGy. Note that the position of the 50% isodose line demonstrates significant compression away from the brain stem and towards the target volume border.

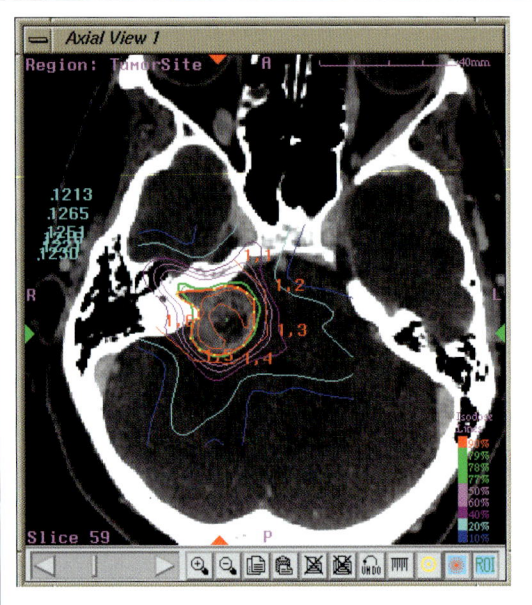

Figure 7. Open curve constraint with marked reduction of the 50% dose to the brain stem.

Method 3. Draw and deposit 3D surfaces which act as a barrier or constraint to beam trajectories passing through critical structures. (CyberKnife users have termed these surfaces "tuning structures.") Tuning structures are manually drawn by the operator in the same manner as any other region of interest.

Figure 8 shows an open curved barrier drawn around the anterior, medial, and posterior aspects of the target and assigned a dose of 1700 cGy. As with the open curve constraint, this barrier also results in compression of the 50% dose away from the brain stem.

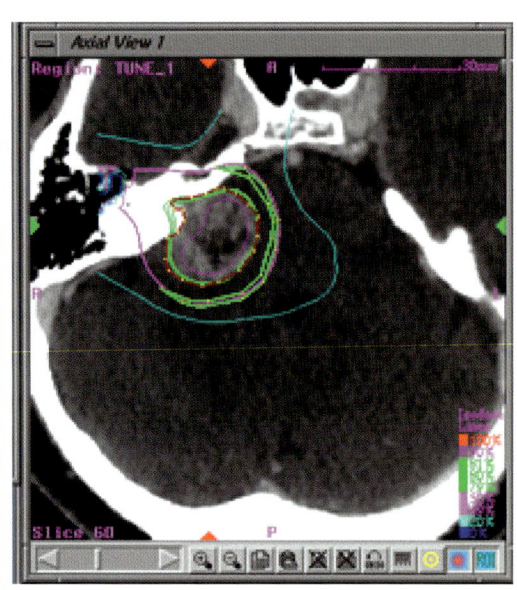

Figure 8. "Tuning structure" constraint with marked reduction of the 50% dose to the brain stem.

Method 4. Expand the target volume by creating a shell around the target volume, by either:

a) Drawing what is termed a soft boundary around the target volume, or

b) Using the auto-expand menu function to create a series of volumes around the target volumes that can be defined at specific distances from the border of the target volume and assigned constraining doses. The autoexpand is useful for limiting the dose in all dimensions surrounding a target volume such as a metastatic lesion within eloquent cortex. However, this could decrease the homogeneity of the dose within the volume.

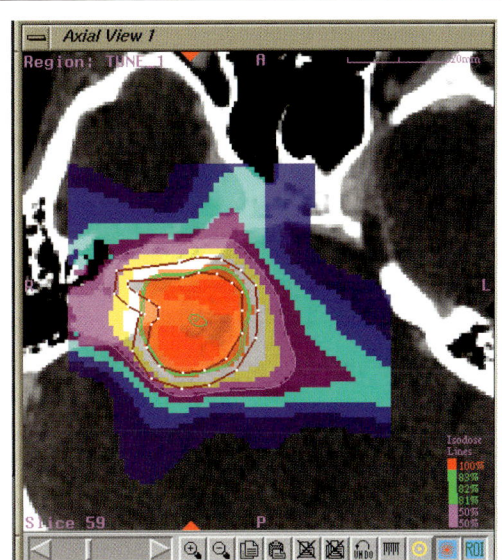

Figure 9. Auto expand target volume boundary resulting in minimal reduction of the 50% dose to the brain stem.

4. Generation of Beam Geometries and Dose Assignment

A. Single and Multiple Isocenter Treatment

Single isocenter treatment planning can be appropriate in the case of a spherical lesion located in a relatively silent area of the brain such as a metastasis in the white matter of the anterior frontal lobe. One might also consider using multiple single isocenters for the treatment of several spherical metastases. This can speed up both the treatment planning process and the treatment delivery time. However, there are very few indications to use multiple isocenters for treatment planning for a single target. An unusual case requiring two or more spherical isocenters would be two or more spherical lesions abutting each other with marked differences in lesion diameters.

Using two isocenters in a single treatment plan with appropriate sized collimators to encompass the two or more contiguous spherical lesions could result in better conformality than using the conformal planning method and could also result in decreased treatment planning and treatment time.

B. Conformal Shape Treatment with Inverse Planning

For the majority of lesions or target volumes the operator should use the conformal treatment shape method to take advantage of the CyberKnife's unique non-isocentric targeting and inverse planning. A significant feature of non-isocentric dose delivery is the ability to use smaller diameter collimators. Although this can cause a relative increase in treatment time, there may be some protective advantage in traversing normal tissue with smaller diameter beams. The most important advantage for using non-isocentric inverse planning is the ability to generate higher homogeneous doses not only throughout the volume of a lesion but particularly in the zone at and within the border of a lesion. Thus, the non-isocentric method is a form of selectively spot welding the target volume.

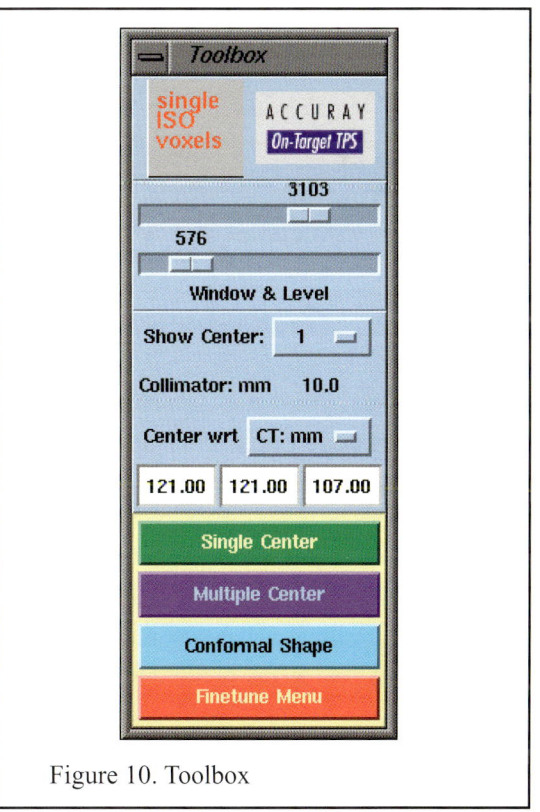

Figure 10. Toolbox

1) Conformal beam assignment

The operator generally starts with a single collimator size that has a diameter approximately 50 to 60% of the narrowest distance across a lesion. Smaller collimators may improve conformality but result in an increased number of beams that could unduly lengthen the time of the treatment. More than one collimator size can be used for a single target volume, but generally this is not necessary.

In the same window the operator also chooses the number of directions for each linac position or node. Generally, one uses all twelve possible directions. The operator can also set the targeting depth inward or outward in millimeters from the outlined border. Figure 11.

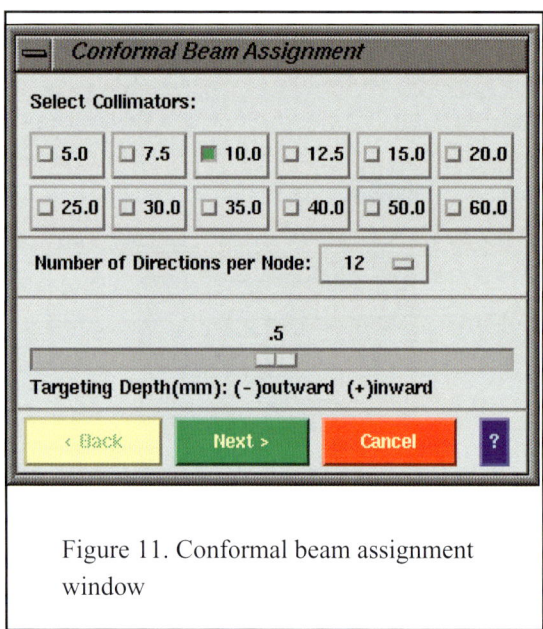

Figure 11. Conformal beam assignment window

2) Conformal dose constraint assignments

There are three ways to attain a conformal dose plan. The most generally used is inverse planning dose assignment. Forward planning is also available, but this method is rarely used. Similarly, bypass dose assignment is available for interrupting completion of the plan but saving the preliminary processes, though this is seldom used. Thus, the operator should select the INVERSE PLANNING button to open the inverse planning dose assignment window which will provide prompts for assigning doses to various volumes.

The operator begins by assigning minimal acceptable doses to the target volumes and maximal acceptable doses to the defined critical structures. In most cases one should also assign a maximal acceptable dose to the target volume. It is not necessary to assign a minimal dose to the critical structures. See Figure 13.

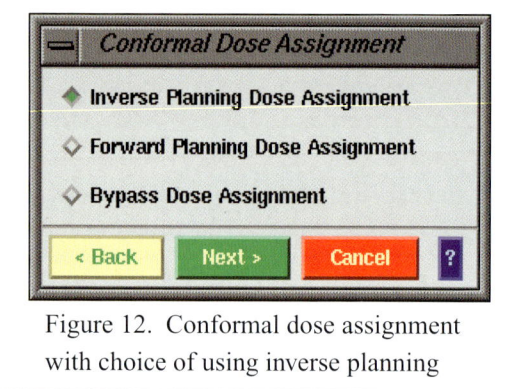

Figure 12. Conformal dose assignment with choice of using inverse planning

3) Target volume dose assignment

Generally, the minimal dose to the target volume is that dose which is 70 to 80% of the maximal dose to the target volume. Note that if one sets no maximal dose, or a maximal dose that is significantly higher than the minimal dose to the target volume, the 80% iso-dose line will be on a steeper portion of the dose response curve. See Figure 13. Theoretically, this could generate a more heterogeneous dose throughout the target volume but a lower dose to an adjacent critical structure.

4) Critical (constraint) structure dose assignment

Assuming that the border of a critical structure is 5 mm or less from the border of the target volume, one begins by assigning a maximal dose to the critical structure that is 50 to 200 cGy below the acceptable dose to the target volume border or the 80% isodose line. If one assigns a maximal dose to a contiguous or close constraint structure that is significantly lower than the acceptable dose to the target volume border, the computation may not be able to generate a solution and will report back in a dialog box on the screen, NO SOLUTION! It is best to start with a dose close to the target volume dose and make certain than a solution can be achieved. Once the computation derives an actual solution, one can repeat the process using a step wise decrease in maximal constraint dose until this manual iteration does not derive a solution. By finding the range of doses between solutions and no solutions, the operator will generally choose the solution that provides the closest maximal critical structure border dose.

5) Limiting constraint numbers

With each added constraint, the time to generate a dose assignment solution increases, and at a certain point the computer will not have access to enough memory to compute a solution. To attain a solution in a practical amount of time initially, one should set the calculation grid in the DISPLAY menu to a COARSE rather than FINE setting. One can then assess whether the total number of constraints seen in the CONSTRAINT SELECTION box is less than 2000. See Figure 13.

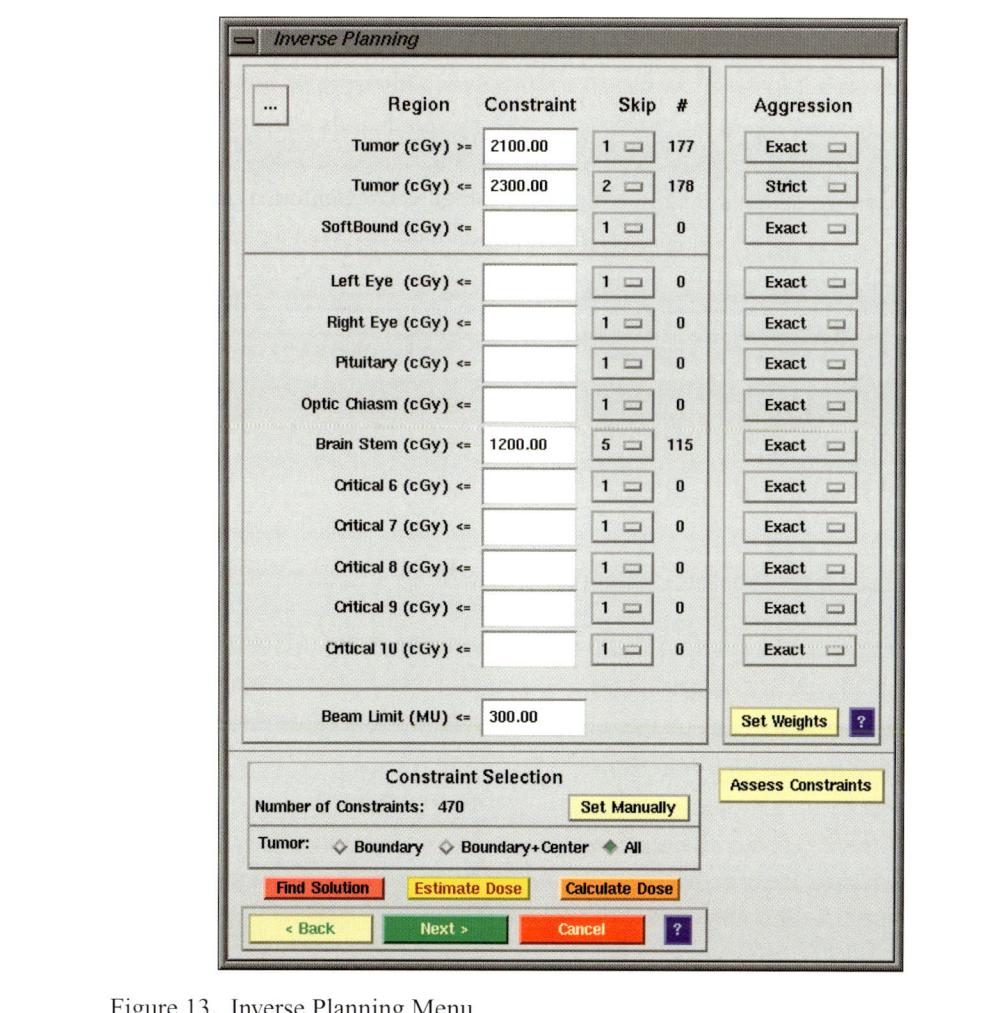

Figure 13. Inverse Planning Menu

The operator can also choose points from 1) the target volume boundary, 2) the target volume boundary and a center point or voxel, or 3) all of the voxels in the target volume. It is best to use the ALL button. In addition the number of constraints for each target volume and critical structure can be adjusted with the SKIP and the AGGRESSION functions. By adjusting these conditions, the number of constraints can be reduced to less than 2000. It is the opinion of the authors of this chapter that making these adjustments to limit the number of constraints does not adversely effect the quality of an acceptable solution. However, each clinician and physicist involved in the radiosurgery prescription must assess personally the quality of each treatment plan that is generated. This assessment is the unique responsibility of the treating physicians.

6) Fine tune menu

The system also provides methods for the operator to add and remove specific beams with the fine tuning menu. There are two methods of accessing the fine tuning menu. The first is through the INVERSE PLANNING menu by accessing the button labeled Set Manually. The second method is by defining manual constraints in the fine tune menu which is accessed through the TOOLBOX menu. With this method the operator adjusts constraints by viewing the trajectory and the assigned dose of specific beams.

The fine tune menu allows the operator to turn on and off individual or groups of beams to improve the conformality of the radiation dose. From a practical point, presently there are two circumstances in which the fine tune menu assists in improving both the solution and the treatment process. If the solution generates individual or groups of beams that are weighted to deliver less than 5 monitor units (mu) or cGy of radiation, then one uses the fine tune menu to turn those beams off. This allows the robot to move the beam more quickly to the next trajectory. If the solution generates a plan that tends to expand the dose of radiation through a portion of a critical structure, some of these clustered beams that generate this dose expansion can be turned off.

One should also be aware that the dose can be impacted by the distance through the air surrounding a body surface to the target volume. A higher than expected radiation dose from a specific beam will be delivered if there is shorter distance through solid tissue to the target volume. Specifically, beams that pass through an air filled sinus such as the maxillary or sphenoid will have higher dose to the target volume which could either positively or negatively impact the conformality of the generated treatment plan. Following each set of changes defined in the fine tune menu, the operator should generate a solution and decide if it is acceptable. Thus, the operator should consider turning off beams if a solution is generated that uses a higher than expected number of beams passing through air sinuses. Likewise, the operator should consider turning off beams in plans for vestibular schwannomas. A somewhat similar consideration occurs when the target volume is close to the brain surface and scalp. Those beams that have a short scalp to target volume distance deliver a higher dose to scalp which may result in a zone of hair loss. By using beams that have a longer distance from the scalp to the target volume, the potential for hair loss can be reduced. However, the operator must weigh whether this beam selection results in the passage of more beams through the brain tissue and possibly critical brain structures. For example, if this type of adjustment results in more dose to the motor cortex or venous structures such as major cortical veins or the sagittal sinus, it would be reasonable to accept the scalp dose rather than brain tissue dose.

7) Set beam limit

By setting a monitor unit (mu) limit, collectively to all of the 1320 possible beams available for a solution, the operator can adjust the solution to utilize a practical number of beams, which depending on the size of the target volume and the collimator size, is generally between 90 and 140 beams. The operator should start with a high beam limit up to 300 mu and reduce it if the solution provides too few beams. This is part of the iteration process with which the operator will gain experience through practice.

8) Find solution process

Once constraint parameters are set, the operator must find a solution. Once a solution is obtained, one can use three different modes to calculate the final dose. One should incrementally increase the number of constraints to find more rigorous solutions. If a solution is not found, one must review the previously described steps to reduce the minimal and maximal dose limits between the target volume borders and the adjacent or contiguous critical structure surfaces and to lower the number of constraints. At a point where the value of the maximal dose limit to the target volume border is close (generally 50cGY or less), a solution will be generated.

5. Dose Calculation

A. Set Calculation Grid

Before the final dose calculations are computed, it is necessary to position and size a grid which represents a cube surrounding the target volume in each of the three views. This cube represents the volume within which the computer calculates the dose. It is positioned by using the cursor to drag its upper right limb in all three views so that it encompasses the target volume and some of the volume of the constraint structures. It is sized by dragging the other borders. This cube also contains cross hairs which should be moved with the cursor in all three views to the relative center of the target volume, if it is a conformal plan, or a specific operator defined iso-center for single or multiple iso-center plans. This calculation grid can then be set to a "coarse" or "fine" mode, which limits the number of voxels involved in the calculation.

The "fine" mode should be used for the final dose calculation. This difference between "coarse" and "fine" can be observed in the number of total constraints after each mode is chosen.

B. Calculate Dose

In each case, no matter which described method is used, once the operator accepts a solution of beam vectors and weighting, the next step is to calculate the actual dose distribution from the selected beams. This is accomplished either by activating the calculate button in the INVERSE PLANNING menu or exiting this menu and moving to the TOOLBOX which will now show a CALCULATION menu in which one can activate either the QUICK CAL solution button or the CALCULATION solution button. The QUICK CAL button calculates only a dose through the coarse calculation grid and only displays the dose in the displayed screen slices. This button is rarely used. Instead, one generally employs the full CALCULATION MODE which provides a dose display through the whole CT study.

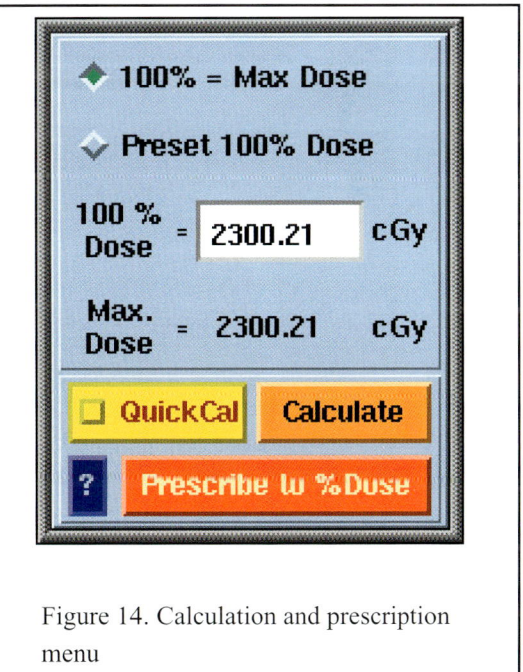

Figure 14. Calculation and prescription menu

C. Saving the Treatment Plan

Once this calculation is completed, the plan should be named, dated, labeled, and saved. A typical label is "arbshape" followed by the size of the collimator, followed by the date the plan was generated, *e.g.*, "arbshape15_11102003." This plan will then be placed in the specific patient's file. When and if one generates additional plans they should be saved with similar but sequential names. Two plans can be compared by bringing up one of the plans in a separate window as a reference plan so that the respective dose distributions can be viewed axial slice by slice.

6. Treatment Plan Assessment

A. Dose Distribution Assessment

1) Isodose curves and point doses

Once the calculation is completed, a set of isodose curves or isodose washes can be overlaid on the 2D image slices. One can assign different numbers of isodose curves with varying percentage values and colors. This allows the operator to view the dose distribution in ways the operator deems appropriate for assessment of the plan. See Figure 15.

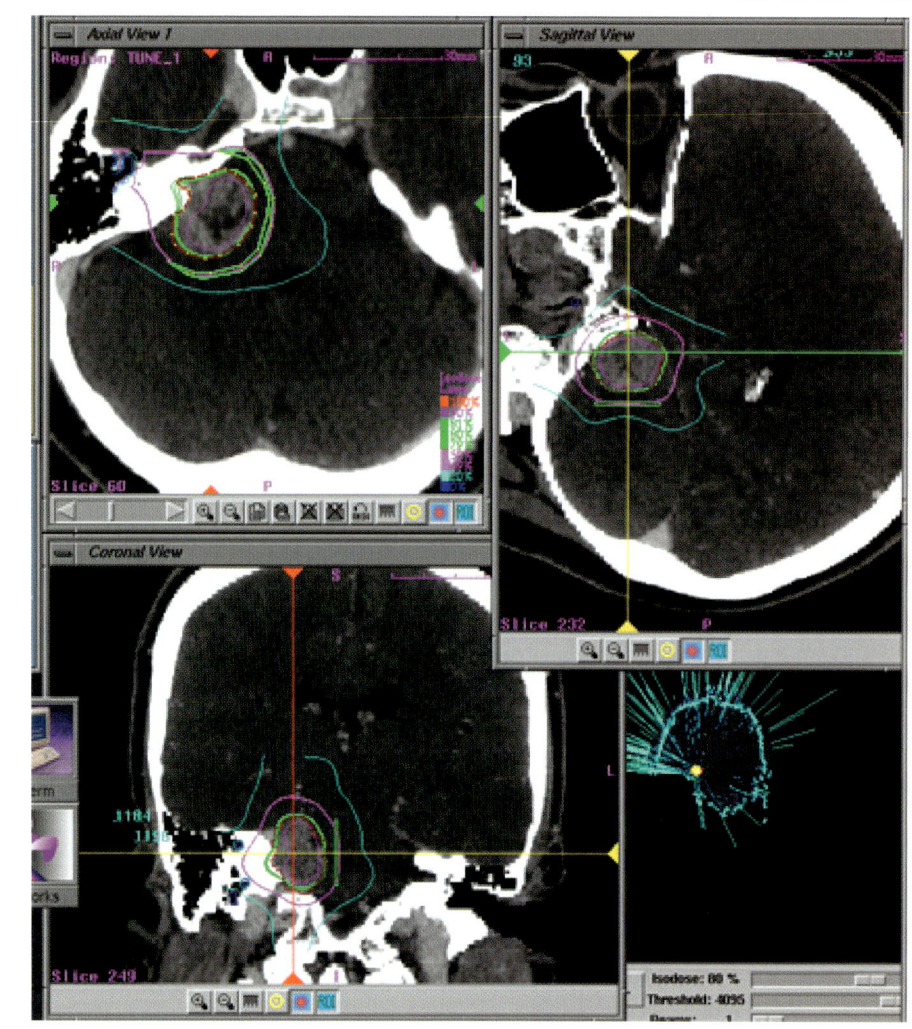

Figure 15. Visual assessment of the isodose curves generated using a tuning structure

Practically, we set one isodose line at 95%, three isodose lines at the prescribed percentage treatment dose to the target volume border which enlarges the width of display of the isodose line prescribed to the target volume border, one isodose line at 50%, and other available lines at the operator's choice. The dose at any point on the anatomy can be viewed by holding down the left mouse button and moving the cursor around the scan image in any of the three views.

2) Dose Volume Histogram and Statistics

The next step is to move to the DISPLAY menu and bring up the dose volume histogram graph (DVH) and the region of interest statistics. One should also view the ASSESS CONSTRAINTS window. These windows provide important graphically and textually displayed information about target and critical structure volumes and the amount of a specific dose encompassing target volume and critical structures.

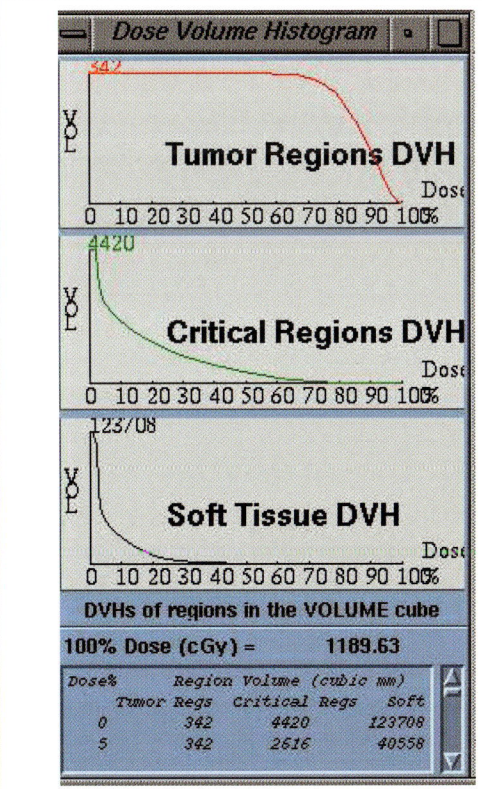

Figure 16. Dose volume histograms and dose statisitcs

B. Plan Summary and Plan Assessment

Lastly, one views the plan summary which displays the number of paths, beams, monitor units, dose in cGy, and non-zero nodes. The plan assessment window allows the tumor dose to be compared to the normal tissue dose. It displays several useful functions including the target volume, the target volume receiving the prescribed dose, volume of critical structures and other normal tissue receiving the prescribed dose. The ratio of total tissue that receives the prescribed dose to the target volume is calculated. This ratio is useful as it describes a conformality index. The closer this ratio is to 1.0, the better the plan protects normal surrounding structures.

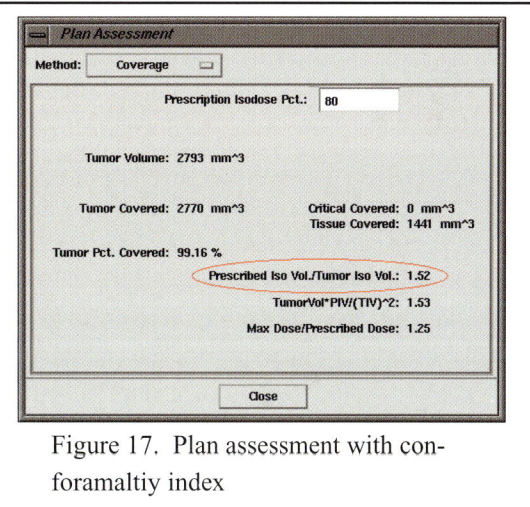

Figure 17. Plan assessment with conforamaltiy index

7. Decision to Treat in More than One Stage or Fraction

If the operator decides that the generated maximal dose to a critical structure is higher than is acceptable, then a plan for staging should be considered. For practical purposes, the determination to stage the treatment occurs primarily in cases in which the border of a critical structure is contiguous or within 5 mm of a target volume border. For example, this type of solution is effective for target volumes adjacent to the optic nerves and optic chiasm and optic tracts, the mid brain and brain stem, and the spinal cord. In all cases, a staging plan can be formulated as follows:

1) Assign a minimal dose to the target volume that is approximately 150 to 200% of the single stage dose.

2) Accept an inversely planned solution that is generated.

3) Divide the maximal computed dose to the critical structure border by the number of stages to define an acceptable dose per stage to that critical structure.

Summary

The CyberKnife treatment planning system expands significantly the capability of delivering highly conformal doses of radiation to asymmetric target volumes. By understanding concepts of non-isocentric beam delivery as contrasted with isocentric beam delivery, one can design treatment plans efficiently by using various constraint mechanisms to maximize dose to the target volume while limiting the dose to surrounding critical structures. With the system's frameless radiographic stereotactic image tracking, one is not limited to single stage treatment. Thus, if a single stage treatment plan results in an unacceptable minimal dose to surrounding critical structures, one can stage the treatment using two or more daily treatments by both increasing the cumulative dose to the target volume and simultaneously limiting the daily dose to the critical structures. This potential staging technique adds to the power of radiosurgery by maintaining ablative conformal doses to target volumes while taking advantage of the protective potential of fractionation or divided dose delivery.

CyberKnife Setup and Treatment

Laurence Jang

Introduction

If you have experience in immobilization devices, setups for CyberKnife should not be difficult, provided that a few rules are followed. If this is your first experience with immobilization without the frame screwed into the patient's head, you'll find there are many different manufacturers of immobilization devices. Generally most of the CyberKnife immobilization devices come from radiation therapy departments. You may chose to use a thermoplastic mask material for your head and neck patients, a vacuum type bean bag or chemical mixed foam mold for extra-cranial patients, or, if need be, some homegrown immobilization device, and even a combination of any of the above devices.

When preparing CyberKnife patients for set-ups, there are many parameters to keep in mind, such as:

Reproducibility. The initial setup table or treatment couch should match the CT table as closely as possible. Variation between the two can result in reproducibility errors and misadministration of dose.

Patient comfort. The patient should be in a position which is comfortable enough to maintain for 45 minutes to 1 hour or more depending on the plan.

An uncomfortable patient who is constantly moving during treatment can degrade accuracy. Remember, the robot corrections are not "real time corrections" but are corrections in between beams or "nodes" depending on the intervals of your image acquisitions.

Artifact. Immobilization devices which interfere with CT or imaging are not appropriate and should not be used.

Patient jewelry should always be removed. Also, removable metallic dental work which could interfere with visualization of a cervical spine level lesion should be removed.

Robot space versus patient space. To avoid creating a hazardous condition, it is imperative to be aware of the space parameters!

Robot space will be defined by your treatment plan and the parameters inputted by the Accuray engineers upon your install. The robot does not have sensors to prevent it from contacting patients. Therefore, the patient should be as flat and compact as possible, with head and arms as close to the table as possible. Any deviation from the original setup could result in collisions, *e.g.*, patients with elevated head and arms, or with arms or elbows extended into robot space will increase the chance of collisions. For the same reason, furniture, objects or medical devices other than those permanently installed by Accuray must not be left near the robot.

Medical problems and allergies. Will the patient need pharmaceuticals during treatment? All the immobilization devices in the world will not help if your patient has back problems, arthritis or claustrophobia problems, to name a few. Observe the patient and ask questions during setups to plan for any potential problems during treatments.

Make sure patient has been screened according to your institution's guidelines. Any potential medical or allergy problems may require patient to be pre-medicated or scheduled to have an MRI performed after CT for image fusion.

Setup Procedure for Cranial Lesions

Patients with intracranial lesions for CyberKnife treatment at Stanford take the following steps for setups.

Patient should be NPO for four hours before arrival in the department. If not previously completed at consultation appointment, patient fills out contrast and screening consent form for CT. An intravenous access line is placed for contrast injection and any sedation or premedication per each institution's protocol for management of allergic reactions.

Setup personnel are notified, patient is placed on setup or treatment table and immobilization device is created. At Stanford we use the Med-Tec Accuform cushion for the back of head, 4 layers of small cell bubble wrap for additional comfort and as shims for possible mask shrinkage. All these steps go beyond a normal radiation therapy setup. However the extra cushion allows more time for the patient to be comfortable and remain stationary during treatment. Patient should be positioned as close to the center of the CT gantry as possible.

Know your tumor location. Pay close attention to head tilt positions if treating and scanning patients with cervical spine lesions or low cranial lesions. Dental fillings can obliterate cervical spine images. Tilt the head to avoid obscuring tumor locations. Ensure area being treated can be positioned over the detectors. After the cushion for the back of head has been made, the thermoplastic mask is constructed. While shaping the mask to the patient, pay close attention to the nose. A tight mask on the nose will cause your patient some pain and may result in movement. The mask should remain on patient's head for at least 10 minutes after creation to decrease amount of mask shrinkage.

Patient is accompanied to CT by the setup personnel. Patient must be placed on the CT table in the exact configuration as when the mask was made. Appropriate modifications to the CT couch may be necessary to achieve this goal. Doing otherwise may make treatment difficult or impossible if head is scanned in a different position. The newer treatment couches have limited leeway in accommodating changes, however this should not be counted on to compensate for couch and setup differences between CT and treatment.

Before patient is scanned, contrast is used to enhance structures to be treated. Care must be taken in order to use correct scanning parameters. At present the T.P.S. cannot handle more than 300 slices. For intracranial scanning there must be at least 1 cm of space between the superior border of the skull and the superior top slices. The field of view should be centered from ant to post and the scan should cover the entire head. See Accuray's manual for the official parameters. We generally use 1.25 mm slice thickness. All slices must be of the same thickness. Check CT scan before allowing patient to leave. Verify that enough information is available on the CT to do treatment planning. On low quality CT scans tumors might not be visible in which case an MRI may be needed   At Stanford we use a high resolution 16 detector GE light speed CT scanner and rarely need to use MRI.

Patient scan series are transferred over the hospital network to the treatment planning station. Scouts are not needed for treatment planning.

CyberKnife Cranial Treatment

Before the patient enters the treatment room, the patient is advised treatments could take as long as 45 minutes to 1 hour or more on the couch. Patient should be asked if they need to use the toilet. At some time before this point, preferably at the initial setup appointment, the patient's fitness to remain on the couch for the extended period of time should have been determined. Some points which should have been considered are:

Is patient having any back pain?

Any claustrophobia problems?

Incontinence issues.

Excess coughing or sneezing.

Allergies.

Medication issues.

Chills.

Anything relevant to the situation.

Some problems may be taken care of with medications. Be sure that any medications have had adequate time to achieve their desired effects.

Patient is escorted onto the treatment couch and placed in the exact position as when the C.T. scan was done. Doing otherwise can lead to radical couch angles and the inability to fully correct for the patient's position. Ensure patient is comfortable on couch and that the mask is comfortable. The tightness of the mask may be adjusted by varying the amount of layers of bubble-wrap or shims under the patient's head. Remember a comfortable patient translates to a more cooperative patient. Explain treatment procedure to patient. Ask patient to keep their eyes closed. This will help minimize patient movement during treatment.

Bring patient into range of detectors using the pendent controls. First, raise the couch vertically, and then move the couch horizontally into superior position, always checking the clearance between the couch, detectors and patient. Any bumping of the couch into the detectors is an immediate cause for concern. If this occurs, treatment should stop immediately and recalibration of imaging detectors must be performed.

Ensure couch is in original setup position before taking images. Take images of patient and adjust accordingly to the imaging system. We generally take out couch shifts first before correcting for rotations.

Always visually compare images for rotation and shift corrections, because noise may cause false readings. For example, the system may show a rotation, which may not be valid and also could show no rotation needed when, in fact, a rotation is needed.

Generally when starting treatment the shifts or robot corrections should be less than 1 mm and less than 1 degree, if possible. Always visually check patient to verify robot corrections.

During treatment always and continuously monitor patient, robot, and treatment system. Make adjustments as necessary.

CyberKnife Extra-Cranial Setup

Screen patients as for cranial patients.

Fiducials placed by surgeons should always be Accuray approved. Accuray should be consulted in advance of treatment if not using approved fiducials.

For patients with gold seeds or wires there should be at least one week between placement of fiducials and setups to allow for migration of fiducials. If fiducials migrate between setup date and treatment date, they will become useless and inaccurate. With screws, setups can be done as soon as patient is able to tolerate the procedure, provided there is no significant swelling in the screw placement area.

Construct immobilization device keeping in mind that, for extra-cranial lesions, the risk of patient collision with the robot increases. Head and shoulders should remain as flat as possible. Depending on location of the target area, arms may need to be positioned above the head. A vacuum bag or alpha cradle may be used to immobilize patient. If necessary, place arms above the head and as flat as possible to minimize beams through unnecessary tissue. Keep in mind patient will also need to fit through the CT scanner. When doing so, allow support for arms while keeping them low enough to stay out of robot space to avoid collisions. The patient's arms may become sore during treatment. Some patients may require pauses during treatment for arm rest or arm repositioning.

For lower cervical and upper thoracic lesions, the neck and shoulders should be stabilized.

If possible, construct the immobilization device in a therapy setup room.

Mark the center of the fiducials on the patient and index it to the immobilization device.

Mark the laser crosshairs on both the immobilization device and the patient both on the CT table and the treatment table for reproduciblity and to minimize setup time.

For gated breathing treatments with pancreas, lung or any other organ which moves with breathing, the patient should be instructed and advised to practice at home breath holding prior to the set up date. During the CT scan, if the patient can hold their breath for the entire scan (usually 35-40 seconds on G.E. Lightspeed 16 I scanner), the DRR's will be more accurate.

Scan patient centering the study on the region of interest. Again, image up to 300 slices with the field of view encompassing all of the patient's anatomy that surrounds the region of interest. All slices must be of the same thickness. Use contrast if necessary. Anterior-posterior and lateral x-ray scouts should be used to insure complete coverage with the CT.

CyberKnife Extra-Cranial Treatment

Screen patient as for cranial patients also checking into patient's physical and toilet needs as treatments can be prolonged. Patient should be NPO for treatment or have a very light meal prior to treatment. With extra-cranial patients, depending on the area being treated, it may be advisable to administer anti-emetic medication prior to and after treatment.

Position patient as with cranial instruction except using fiducial tracking. Use marks placed on patient and center them over the detectors. Use similar instructions and screening as for cranial patients. Warn the patient that the robot will come close and the operators will be monitoring if the robot is too close to the patient.

Know your robot space and patient space.

Always monitor patient, robot and tracking system. A dangerous situation could exist if the robot collides with patient. Always be ready to pause or stop robot during treatment. Constantly monitor tracking making sure correct fiducials are being tracked. If corrections radically change during tracking, system should be stopped and patient re-imaged. Occasionally the robot can block the imaging system, which can cause tracking errors.

Occasionally patients may need to periodically rest their arms during treatment.

For patients who may have extended treatment times an airbag or massaging boot may be placed around patient's legs to prevent any chance of deep venous thromboses.

If using breath-holding techniques, always determine patient's breath holding capabilities at setups. It may take a while to build up patient's breathing pattern.

Conclusion

Setups and treatments for CyberKnife will become increasingly more complex as treatments are expanded to other parts of the body. Keep an eye open for new and improved immobilization devices and techniques that can be incorporated into treatment methods.

Fiducials for Target Localization

Derek Olender

Introduction

For treating lesions outside the skull, the CyberKnife system uses radiographic markers for target localization. This chapter will explore the process by which these fiducials are identified and tracked as well as the techniques employed by the operator to assist the system in accurately defining the fiducial locations.

Treatment delivery using fiducial markers is accomplished by comparing the locations of the markers identified in two-dimensional live treatment radiographs to locations of the same markers identified in the treatment CT during treatment planning. Analysis involves a two step process that includes identification of fiducials in the live images (fiducial extraction) and a comparison of their positions against the fiducials in DRRs generated from the CT (correlation). When fiducial extraction occurs without error, correlation is automatic; if extraction fails, no correlation will occur.

When used correctly, fiducials can assist the user in delivering treatments with sub-millimeter accuracy. The accuracy of the treatment delivery, however, is dependent on several factors. First, when using fiducials, certain criteria must be satisfied. First, the fiducial body (the volume created by all fiducials being tracked) must be rigidly fixed to a location in the body, and this volume must be static with relationship to the lesion being treated. Second, fiducials and their locations must be accurately identified by the Target Localization System (TLS). We will explore methods to ensure that the system properly identifies and tracks the fiducial markers.

Limitations of Fiducial Tracking

Fiducial tracking can provide highly accurate treatment delivery. However, failure to understand the limitations of this system can cause reduced accuracy or tracking failure.

1. Use of Approved Fiducials

Currently, there are two types of fiducials approved by Accuray for use with the CyberKnife system. While unapproved fiducial markers may be recognized by the image guidance system, using such fiducials may present difficulties for consistent fiducial identification and tracking. Use of approved fiducials is recommended. The two types of fiducials approved for use are steel screws and gold seeds. The steel screws, intended for bony applications, are distributed through Accuray. For soft tissue applications, gold seeds are available from MedTec or Alpha-Omega.

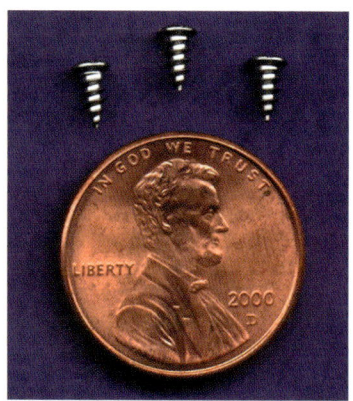

Figure 1. 2.0 mm x 5.0 mm steel radiographic marker screws

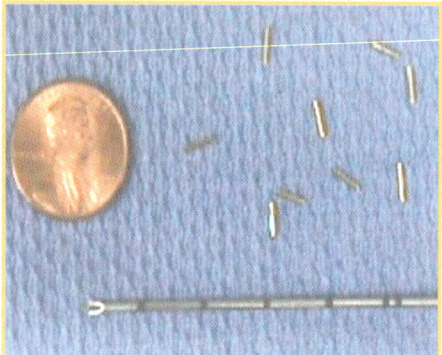

Figure 2. 1.25 mm x 5.0 mm gold seeds by MedTec

Geometric Constraints

To accurately track fiducials in 6 dimensions (three translations and three rotations), fiducial configurations must meet certain minimum requirements. The location of fiducials, determined by the surgeon placement, will affect the system's ability to accurately track fiducials.

The number of fiducials being tracked has a direct effect on tracking accuracy. To calculate translational movements only, it is necessary to track only one fiducial. Translational tracking accuracy improves, but at a diminishing rate, as more fiducials are used. If the operator wants to track patient rotations in addition to translations, a minimum of three fiducials must be tracked. As with translational accuracy, rotational accuracy also improves as the number of fiducials increases. The total error in patient pose (a combination of translations and rotations) is also dependent on the number of fiducials being tracked, but tracking more than six fiducials does not offer significant improvements in accuracy (1). Therefore, it is recommended that four to six fiducials be tracked.

In addition to being dependent on the number of fiducials being tracked, accuracy is also affected by the geometry of the fiducial configuration. In order for the CyberKnife system to track rotations, two minimum geometric constraints must be met. First, fiducials must not be colinear if the system is to calculate rotations. In the Treatment Delivery System (TDS), there is a "Colinearity Threshold" of 15 degrees. This value specifies that there must be an angle of at least 15 degrees between any two fiducials before the system will calculate rotations. This constraint can be reduced by the operator, but doing so will reduce the accuracy with which the algorithm is able to calculate rotations.

In addition to the colinearity constraint, there is also a "Fiducial Spacing Threshold" constraint of 2.0 cm. This value defines the minimum distance between fiducials if they are to be considered for rotational calculations. There must be at least three fiducials in the configuration that satisfy this constraint if the application is to calculate rotations. As with the colinearity constraint, this value, too, can be reduced, but doing so will reduce fiducial tracking accuracy (Fig. 3.).

In summary, the most accurate fiducial tracking will be achieved if the operator is able to track 4 to 6 fiducials placed at least 2.0 cm apart with an angle of not less than 15 degrees between fiducials.

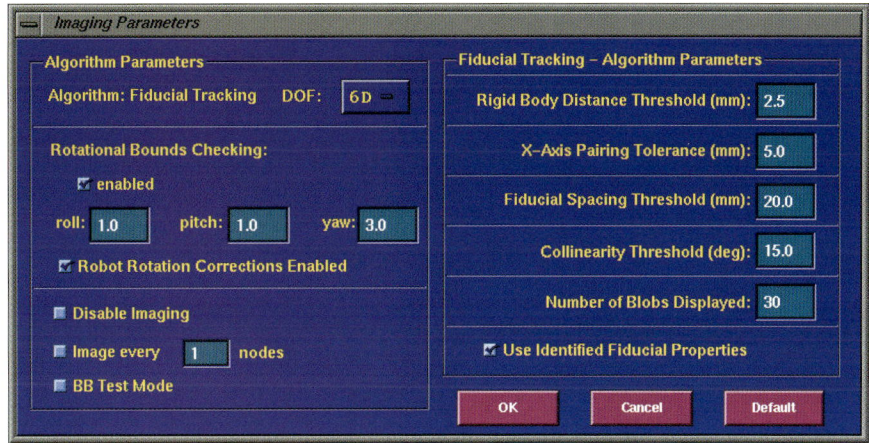

Figure 3. User adjustable constraints for spacing and co-linearity can be adjusted in the *Imaging Parameters* window

Principles of Fiducial Extraction

A basic overview of the principles of fiducial extraction and correlation is warranted. Understanding this process will assist the user in making appropriate interventions throughout the extraction and treatment processes.

The first step in fiducial extraction involves thresholding the live radiographic images to produce white on black images (Fig. 4). In each extraction, the region being searched is processed multiple times at different threshold values to create a library of threshold examples. Areas of white on black (referred to as "blobs") in these threshold exposures are compared throughout the library, and those with the same location in each example are assumed to be the same object. The number of appearances (n) of each blob is counted (Fig. 5).

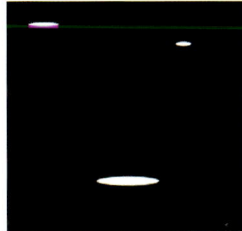

Figure 4. Example of threshold for fiducial extraction

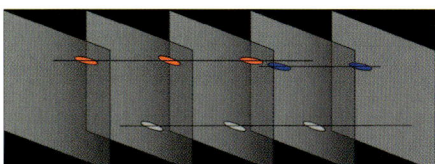

Figure 5. Blobs with similar locations in different threshold exposures are counted as multiple appearances of same object

In the second step, the TLS reduces the number of occurrences of each blob from n to 1 and ranks them in order of likelihood of being a fiducial. This is accomplished by comparing all the examples for the blob against a set of predefined characteristics that include shape, size, and exposure levels. The example of the blob that most closely matches the expected characteristics is identified as the "blob of best fit," and its characteristics are retained as the defining characteristics for the blob. In this step, blobs that don't match the expected characteristics are discarded. The remaining best fit blobs are then ranked by the TLS in the order that their characteristics fit the expected parameters, creating a hierarchy of blobs most likely to be fiducials.

The third step in fiducial extraction is to create three-dimensional potential fiducials from the two two-dimensional blobs. Blob locations in the two live radiographs are compared against the inferior-superior axis of the patient. Those blobs that have corresponding positions in the two images are assumed to originate from the same object in the patient, and the location of this object can be calculated in three-dimensions by projecting backward from the two images. These two blobs are now considered a single fiducial candidate.

In the final step of the fiducial extraction, the TLS creates a fiducial configuration from all the potential fiducial candidates. To execute this step, the TLS compares all the potential configurations created by all the fiducial candidates against the reference configuration in the Treatment Planning System (TPS). Any configuration that does not match the expected configuration is discarded. Those that match the configuration are ranked according to best fit and highest quality fiducials until only one configuration remains. From this configuration, individual fiducials can be identified. It is important to understand that the entire configuration must pass for any of the fiducials within it to be considered. Therefore, if one fiducial in the configuration fails the extraction process, the entire configuration will fail, a fact that has direct implications in the patient tracking and treatment delivery process.

Using Fiducials for Treatment Delivery

There are two methods of fiducial tracking to assist the user in positioning and treating the patient. The first method is "Search." In the Search mode, the TLS searches the live radiograph from each camera for the entire fiducial array. This method is useful when trying to grossly position the patient within the bounds of the imaging system. Search mode is dependent on the successful extraction of all fiducials within the patient. In cases where one or more fiducial is obscured or difficult to identify, the Search function will not give the user the feedback necessary to reposition the patient. When the search mode fails, it may be necessary to use the second method for fiducial tracking.

The second method for tracking fiducials is the "Track" mode in which the TLS searches for each fiducial independently by dividing the live images into Regions of Interest (ROI) corresponding to the expected location for each fiducial. Fiducials that do not fall within their expected ROI in the live images can be misidentified or may fail the extraction process entirely. During initial patient positioning, it is unlikely that all the fiducials will fall within their regions of interest, so additional steps may be necessary to assist the TLS in extracting and identifying the fiducials.

Prior to treatment delivery, the patient must be aligned properly (Fig. 6). In this step, fiducial tracking is used to move the patient into the treatment area within the constraints specified by the user (Fig. 7) and as defined in the limits of manipulator motion. Once the patient is in the treatment position, the TLS can track the patient during treatment delivery. In the sections that follow, a technique for positioning and tracking the patient will be discussed. Individual users may choose to modify this technique based on experience or specific clinical needs on a case by case basis.

1. Patient alignment using the Search mode

The first step in patient alignment is to place the patient on the treatment couch using the appropriate immobilization devices and then to move the couch so that the fiducial body falls roughly in the center of the imaging system. The user need only estimate patient positioning at this point. Once the treatment room is clear, the operator should acquire a live image (Fig. 8) using the Search mode to check patient position. If the TLS is able to extract all the fiducials, it will correlate the patient position and return the couch correction values necessary for positioning the patient more precisely. Known fiducials are marked with green diamonds in the DRR's and the fiducials extracted from the live images are marked with green with green cross-hairs. Couch corrections are calculated by measuring the offset between these two sets of fiducials. If the patient is not within the bounds specified, the application will first warn the user of this fact (Fig. 9). After repositioning the patient, another live image is acquired. This process is repeated until the patient is adequately positioned.

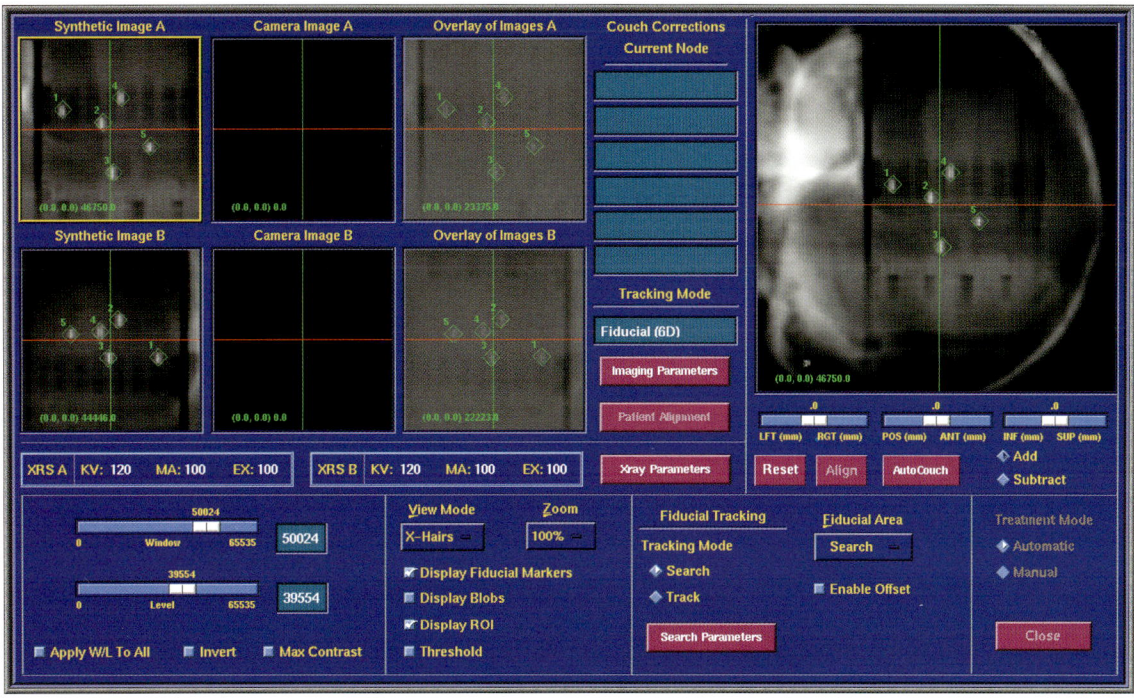

Figure 6. *Patient Alignment* screen in Search mode

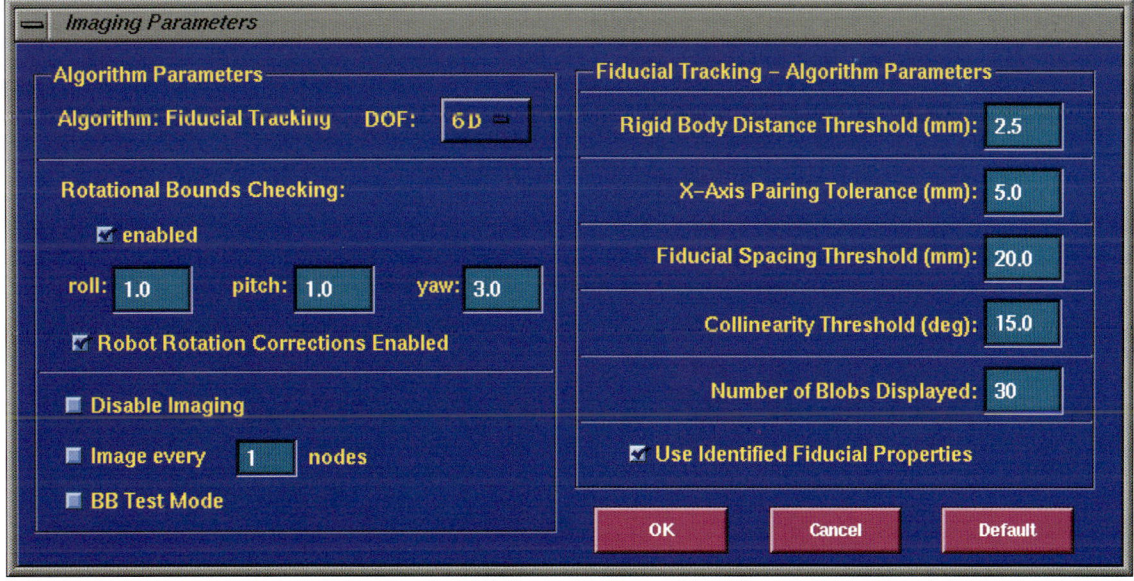

Figure 7. Rotational limits acceptable for patient positioning are specified in the *Imaging Parameters* window

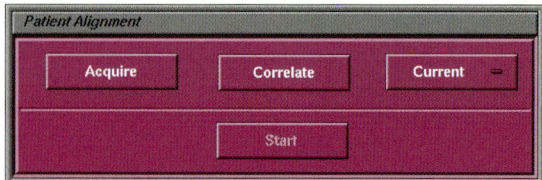

Figure 8. Image acquisition options available during patient alignment

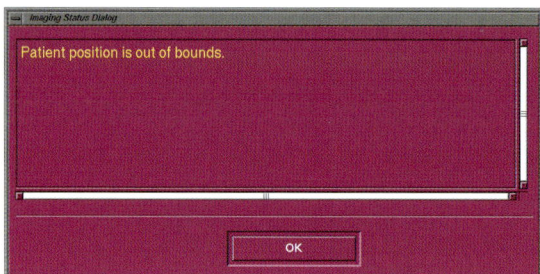

Figure 9. *Patient Out of Bounds* dialog box:

In many cases, not all fiducials can be identified on the first attempt. In such cases, the user will be alerted that the fiducial extraction failed (Fig. 10). When this occurs, it may be necessary to switch the TLS into Track mode.

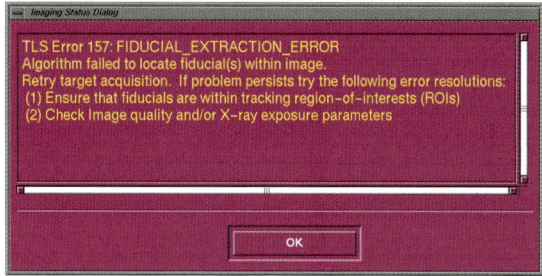

Figure 10. *Fiducial Extraction Error* dialog box

2. Patient alignment using the Track mode

Alternately, some users may find it easier to begin patient alignment using Track mode, bypassing the Search function entirely. In either case, using Track mode gives the operator greater influence over the manner in which the TLS searches for and identifies fiducials (Fig. 11).

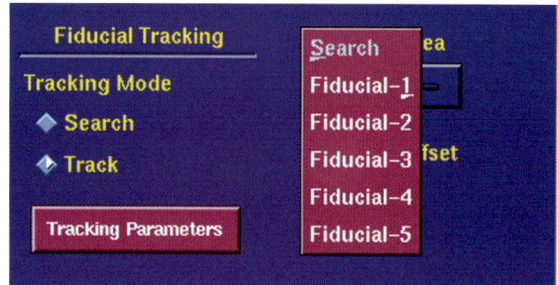

Figure 11. *Patient Alignment* can be finely adjusted in Track mode

After immobilizing and positioning the patient, the operator should acquire a live image in the same manner as described in the above section. In almost all cases, the user will be given a Fiducial Extraction error as in Figure 10. This is due to the fact that the TLS is searching for individual fiducials in very limited ROIs, and very rarely will the operator be able to position the patient so that all the fiducials fall within their expected ROIs. There are two methods available to assist the user in placing the fiducials within their expected ROIs.

Using the "View Mode" drop down menu (Fig 12), the user can select the "Offset" function. This function allows the user to manually reposition all ROIs as a group over their respective fiducials in the live images. This step will force the TLS to search for the fiducials in the newly repositioned Regions of Interest (Fig 13 and 14).

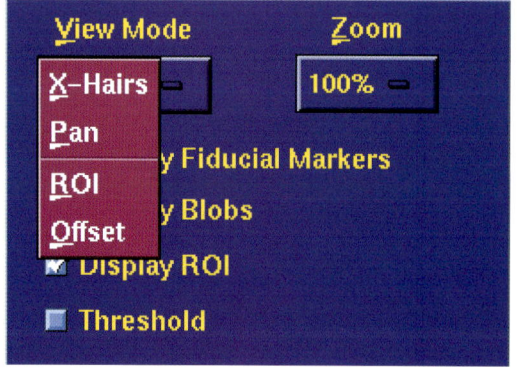

Figure 12. "View Mode" menu

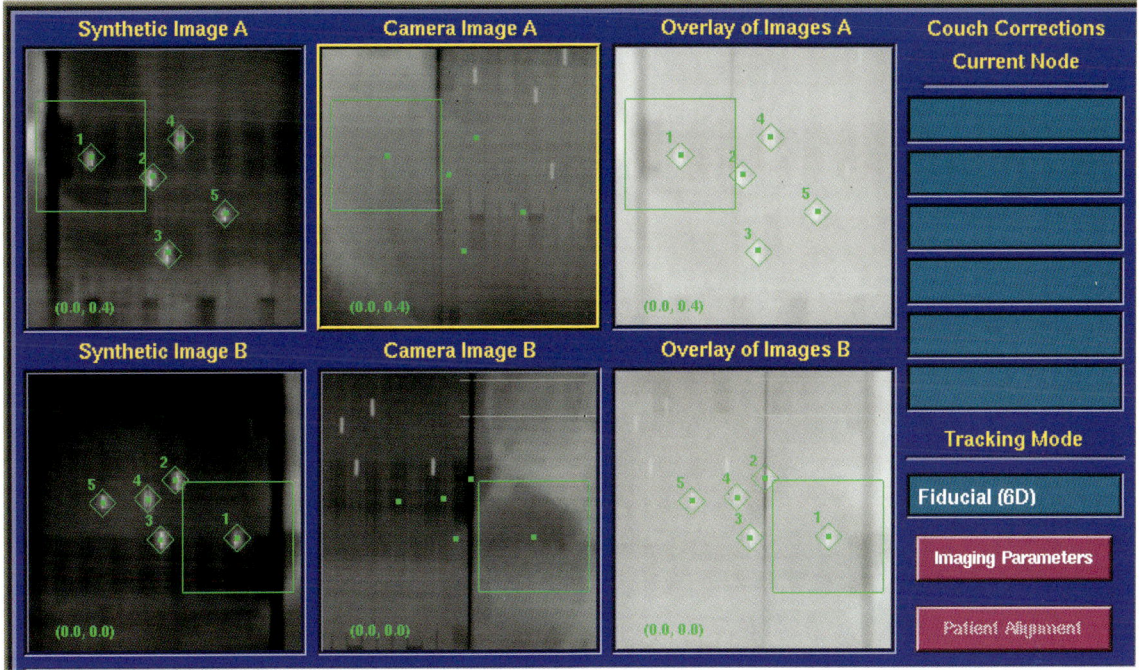

Figure 13. Offset mode showing the expected locations of all fiducials

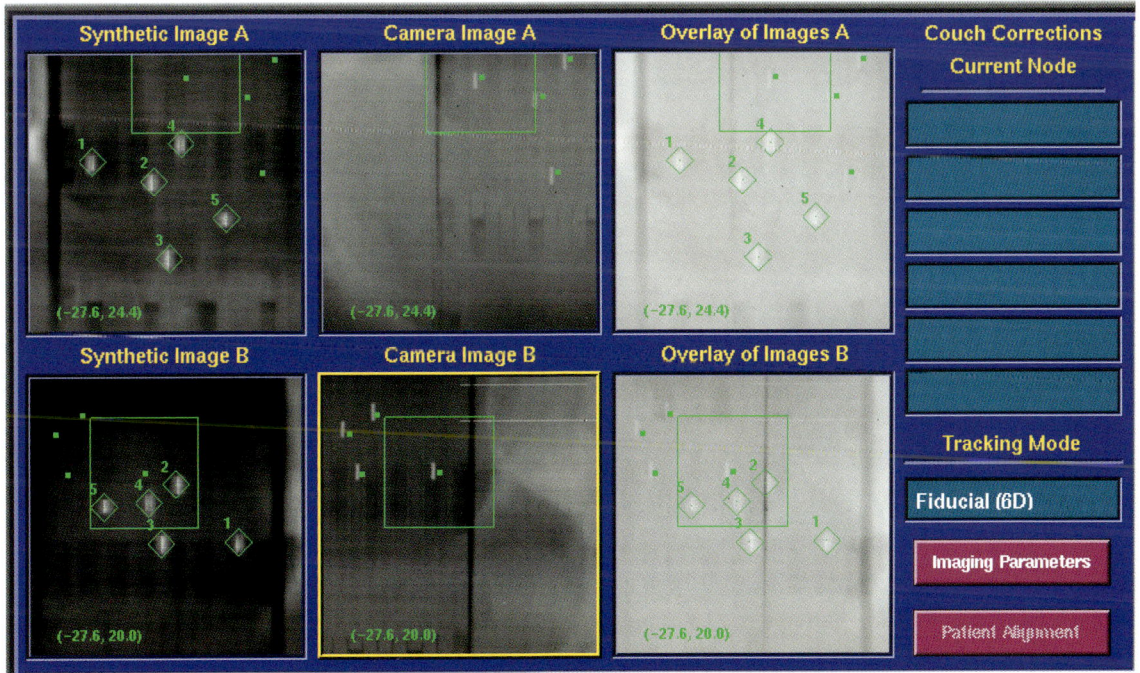

Figure 14. Offset mode after repositioning the ROIs over their respective fiducials

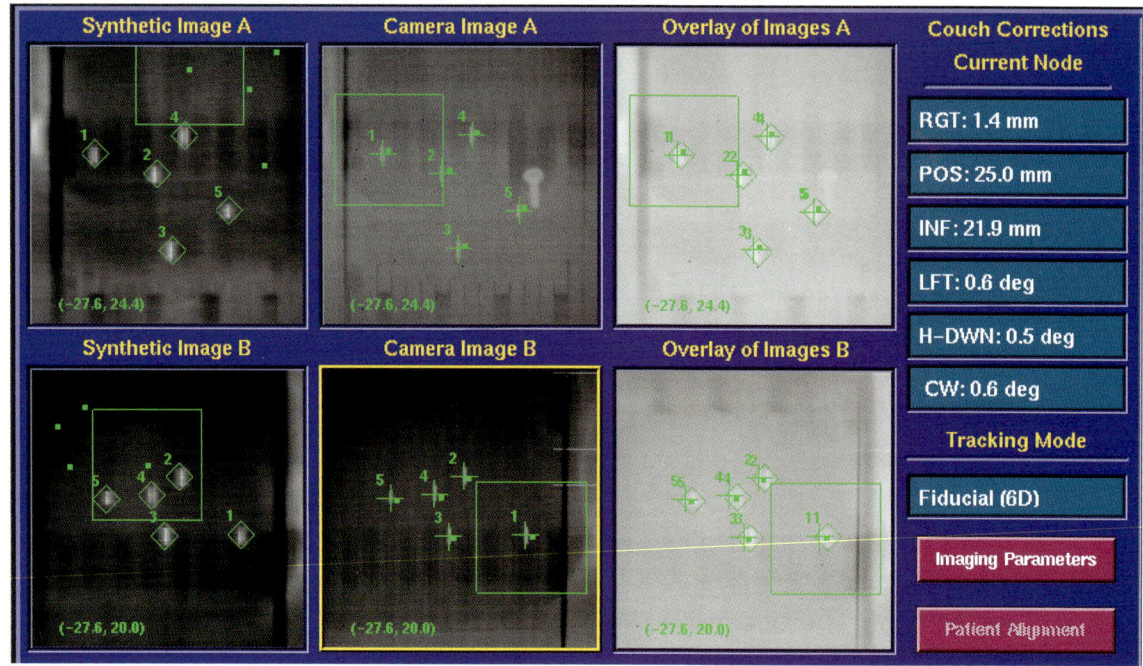

Figure 15. Correlated patient position after using Offsets

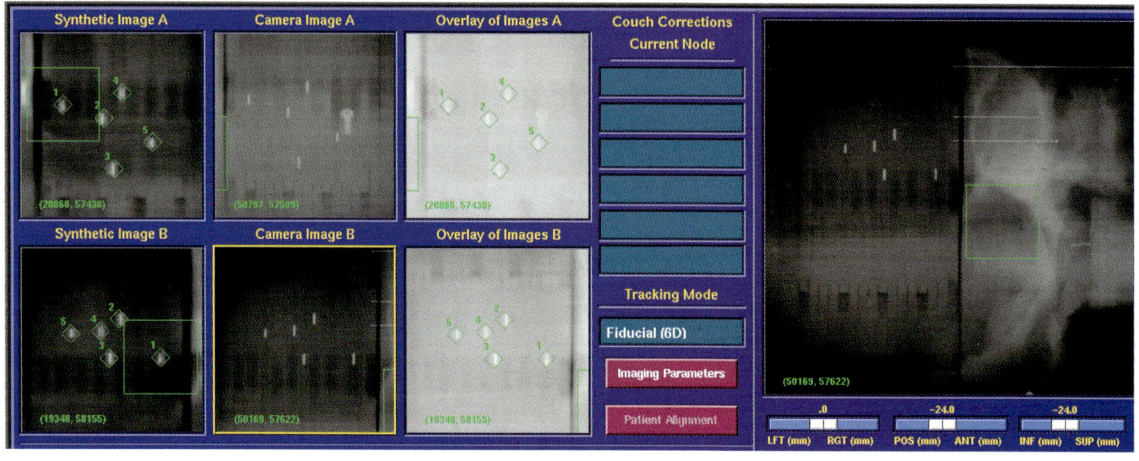

Figure 16. An estimate of couch corrections can be attained using the couch position scroll bars

Once the ROIs are repositioned, it is not necessary to acquire a new set of live images. Instead, the operator can use the "Correlate" button (Fig. 8) to attempt a new fiducial extraction and correlation using the redefined ROIs (Fig. 15). As in Search mode, if the patient falls outside the bounds of proper alignment, the Out of Bounds dialog box will appear before the user sees the updated couch correction values. Once the couch is moved according to these values, another image set can be acquired for additional repositioning.

In situations where the operator does not wish to use the Offset function to move ROIs, patient repositioning can be achieved using the couch position scroll bars to pan the live images. By moving the scroll bars so that the position of the fiducials in the live images corresponds to the position of the fiducials in the DRRs, the user can get an approximation of the couch corrections necessary. Moving the couch by these amounts should bring the fiducials within range of their ROIs once a new set of images is acquired (Fig. 16).

3. Extraction errors during patient alignment

In some cases Search mode, Offsets, and couch positioning will all fail to provide the user with couch correction values because the TLS failed to identify one or more fiducials in the live images. As mentioned earlier, when one fiducial in the configuration cannot be identified, the entire configuration will fail. In these situations, the user will be confronted with a Fiducial Extraction error, regardless of the method employed. It is therefore necessary for the user to identify the problematic fiducial(s) and take steps to assist the TLS with the extraction process.

Identifying problematic fiducials requires a systematic approach by the operator. Failure to approach this problem systematically can lead to a lengthy process of trial and error while the operator attempts to track the problematic fiducial. The easiest means to identify a problematic fiducial is to begin in Track mode with all fiducials turned off for tracking.

In Track mode, the user can see a list of all fiducials under the "Fiducial Area" drop down menu (Fig. 17). Individual fiducials can be selected from this menu, and they can be turned off by deselecting the "Use for Tracking" option of the *Tracking Parameters* window (Fig. 18). Deactivated fiducials will appear as yellow diamonds in the Synthetic images.

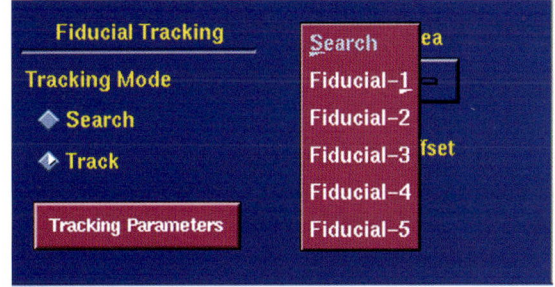

Figure 17. Select individual fiducials from the "Fiducial Area" menu

With all fiducials turned off, the user can acquire a live image and should use this to select one fiducial to start the alignment process. This fiducial should be clearly visible, unobstructed by hardware or anatomy and of good image quality. Begin by reselecting this fiducial for tracking in *Tracking Parameters*. With this fiducial active, select ROI from the "View Mode" drop down menu (Fig. 12). The ROI will most likely miss the location of the fiducial in the live image (Fig. 19).

Using the mouse in the live images, the user can click and drag to draw a new ROI around the fiducial in both live images. Drawing a smaller ROI increases the likelihood that the fiducial will be properly identified, but care should be taken to ensure that the entire fiducial is within the ROI. The new ROI will appear yellow in the live images (Fig. 20). In the *Tracking Parameters* window, select the "Use ROI" button for both cameras. Once this step is complete, the ROI will turn green indicating that it is the active ROI for the fiducial in question (Fig. 21).

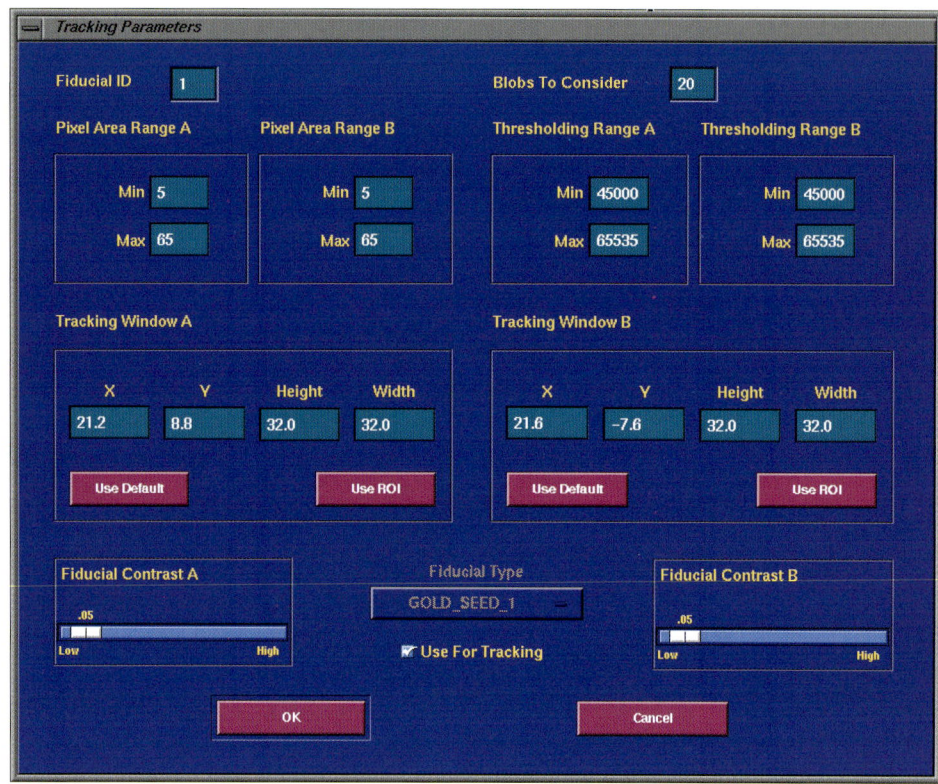

Figure 18. The *Tracking Parameters* window can be used to deactivate/activate a fiducial or to change the search cri-

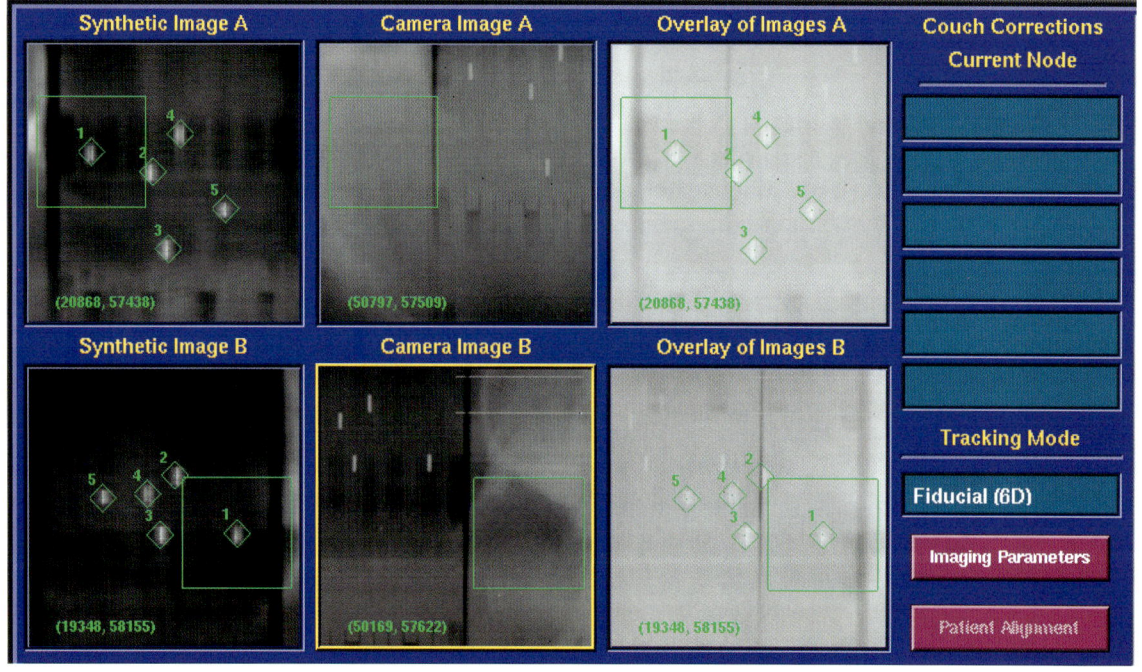

Figure 19. Single fiducial outside its Region of Interest

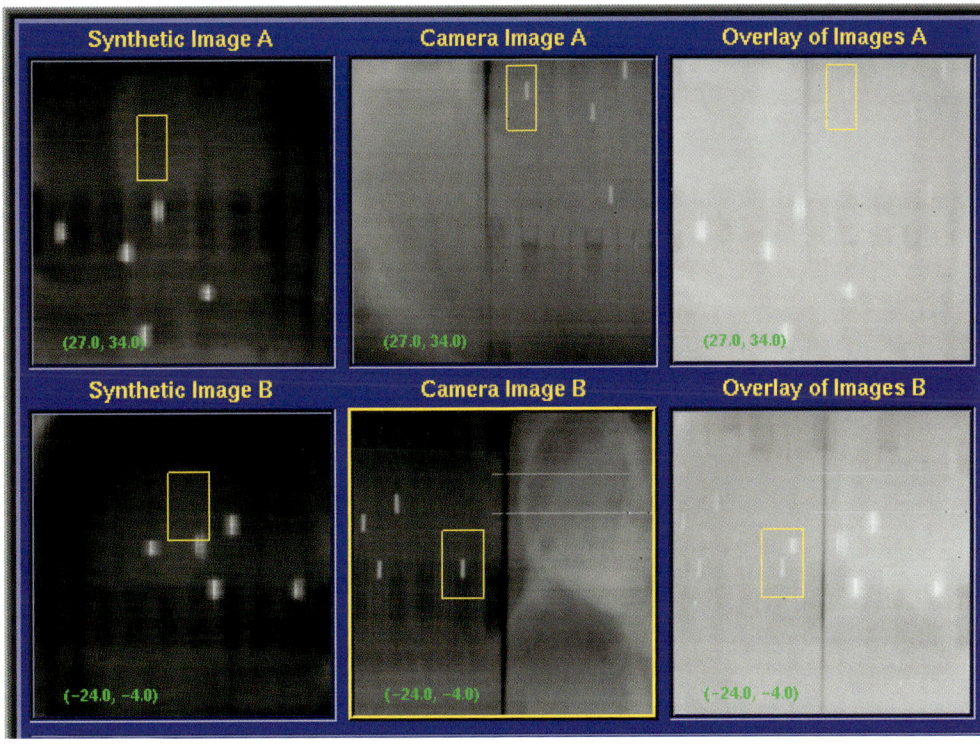

Figure 20. Fiducial within the redrawn ROI

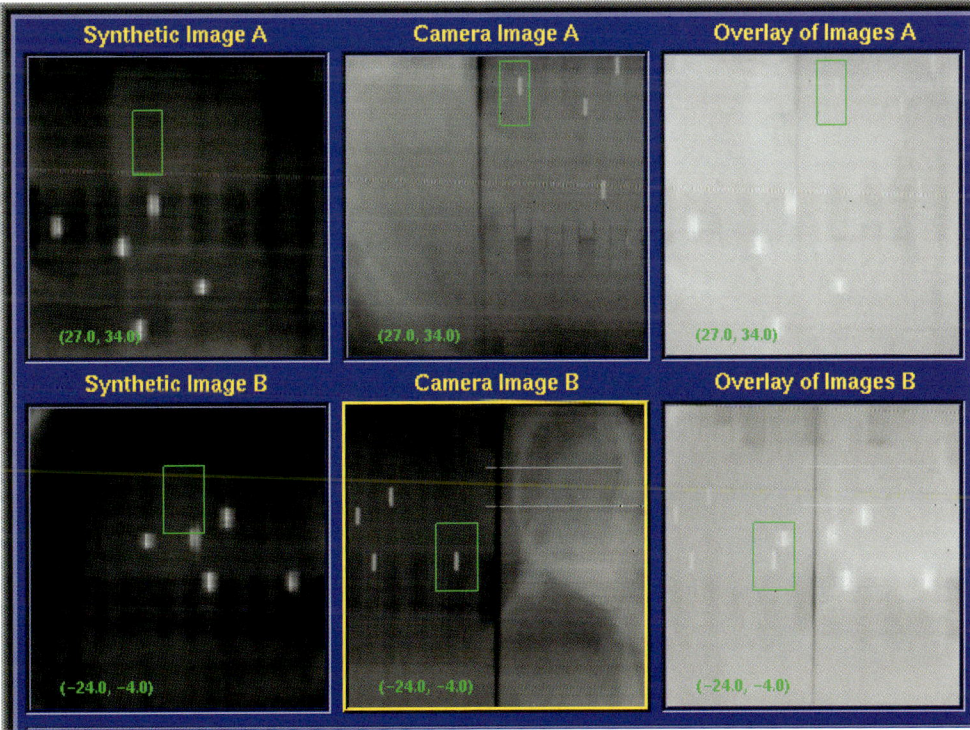

Figure 21. Redrawn ROI turns green once selected from *Tracking Parameters*

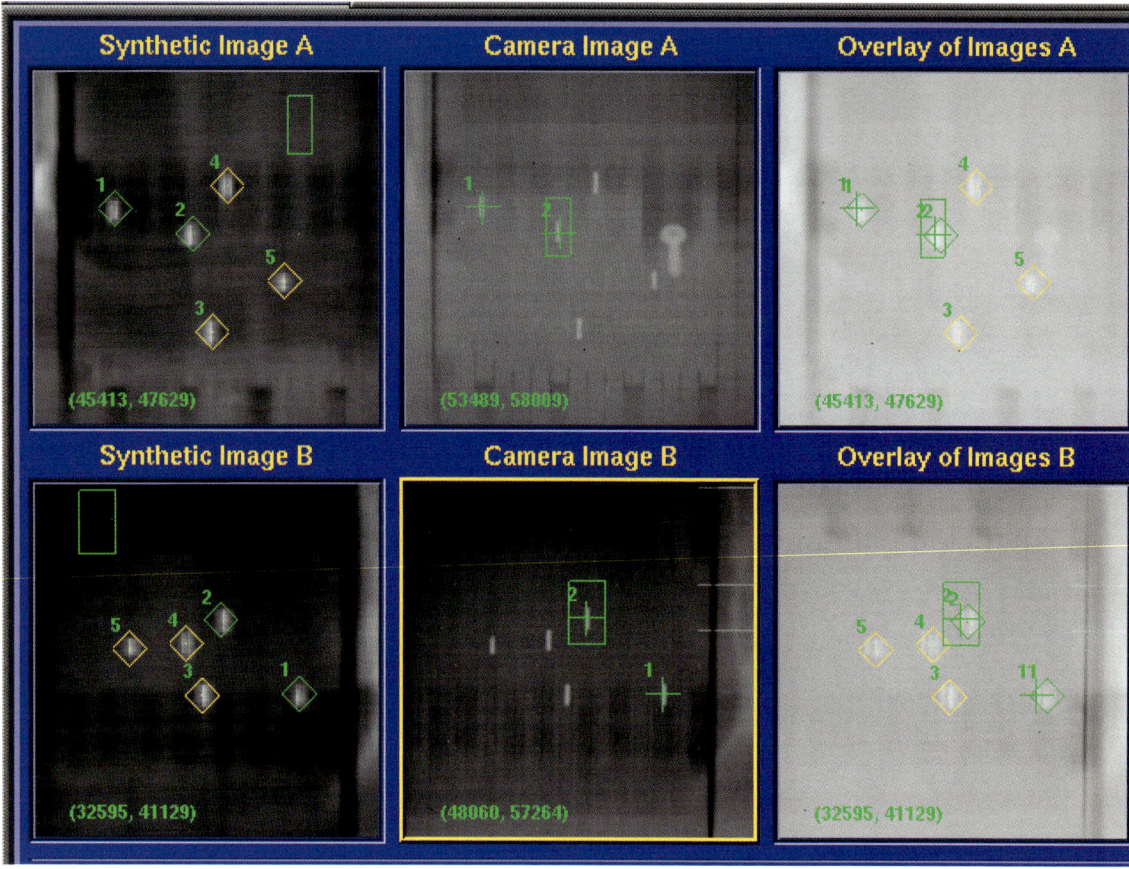

Figure 22. Correlation of image with additional fiducial extracted using drawn ROI. Note the yellow diamonds indicating fiducial not active for tracking

At this point, the operator can select "Correlate" to calculate the patient position using this one fiducial. If correlation is successful, the TLS will give only translational couch corrections since at least three fiducials are required for calculating rotations. Move the couch accordingly.

With the couch in the corrected position, it is necessary to switch from the redrawn ROI to back to the default. Failure to do so will result in the TLS searching in the region where the ROI was drawn previously. Return to the *Tracking Parameters* window and select the "Use Default" button to restore the default ROI. Acquire a new image and verify that the fiducial is properly identified. If not, redraw the ROI again and use the redrawn ROI for further correlations. Make sure that this ROI is large enough so that small patient movements will not move the fiducial outside the bounds of the ROI.

Select another fiducial from the "Fiducial Area" menu and activate it for tracking. Attempt to correlate using the default ROI. If correlation fails, redraw its ROI as with the first fiducial and select "Use ROI" from the *Tracking Parameters* window. Correlate the image with the new ROI (Fig. 22). Repeat these steps with additional fiducials until all the fiducials have been turned on or until identification of a fiducial that cannot be extracted and correlated.

Once the problematic fiducial has been identified, the user has several options. One option is to attempt treatment with the errant fiducial turned off. While doing this may work from a technical standpoint, it may compromise accuracy as noted in the opening section of this chapter.

4. Extraction of difficult fiducials:

In some cases, treating with a problematic fiducial turned off may not be an option. When the increased accuracy provided by an additional fiducial is desired, or if there are not enough fiducials remaining to calculate rotations, the user may wish to pursue attempts to identify this fiducial. First, the user must determine if the fiducial can be extracted at all. This requires several steps. In the *Patient Alignment* window (Fig. 6), select the "Threshold" check box. Adjust the Window and Level scroll bars so that the shape of the questionable fiducial (in white) becomes visible on the black image. Continue to adjust the scroll bar until the fiducial area starts to shrink. The fiducial must become distinct from its surroundings before it disappears. If the thresholded fiducial shape does not separate from its surroundings (hardware, anatomy, etc) before disappearing, extraction will not be possible because it will not get identified as a blob during the thresholding step of the extraction process.

If the thresholded fiducial appears as a distinct, discrete object of white on black, it is very likely that the user will be able to find a way to make extraction successful. Several options are available, the easiest of which is to adjust the x-ray technique to increase contrast in the image. Increase the x-ray techniques in small increments using the *X-ray Parameters* window (Fig. 23). Correlate between adjustments. Care should be taken not to over expose the image, as this may cause the fiducials to wash out and could complicate further extraction.

If adjusting the x-ray technique is not successful, the user can try changing the search parameters used for an individual fiducial. Begin by selecting the "Display Blobs" check box on the *Patient Alignment* window. When "Display Blobs" is selected, the TLS will highlight the two-dimensional blobs that failed consideration as fiducial candidates. If the desired fiducial is not highlighted in a yellow diamond in the live image, increase the value for "Number of Blobs Displayed" in the *Imaging Parameters* window (Fig. 7) until it becomes highlighted.

Once it is highlighted, click on the center of the yellow diamond around the desired fiducial until it becomes blue. In the large image in the alignment window, right mouse click and select to display the Imaging Log. When the blob is selected and marked in blue, its properties will be displayed in the Imaging Log (Fig. 24). Use the displayed values for Pixel Area, Threshold and Contrast to adjust the search criteria found in the *Tracking Parameters* window for the desired fiducial. Select a narrow range for Pixel Area Range and Thresholding Range that includes the displayed values. Select a contrast value just below the displayed contrast for the blob. Attempt to correlate with the new parameters. If correlation fails, adjust the x-ray technique as described above and repeat correlations. If correlations continue to fail, extraction may not be possible.

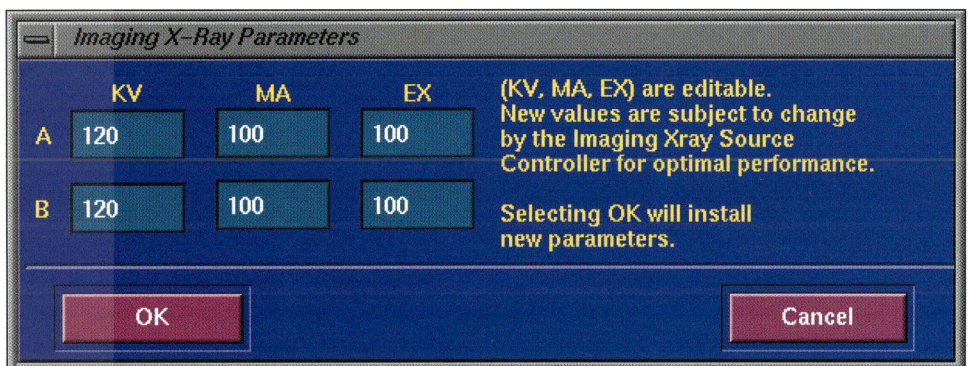

Figure 23. X-ray technique for live images can be adjusted in the *X-ray Parameters*

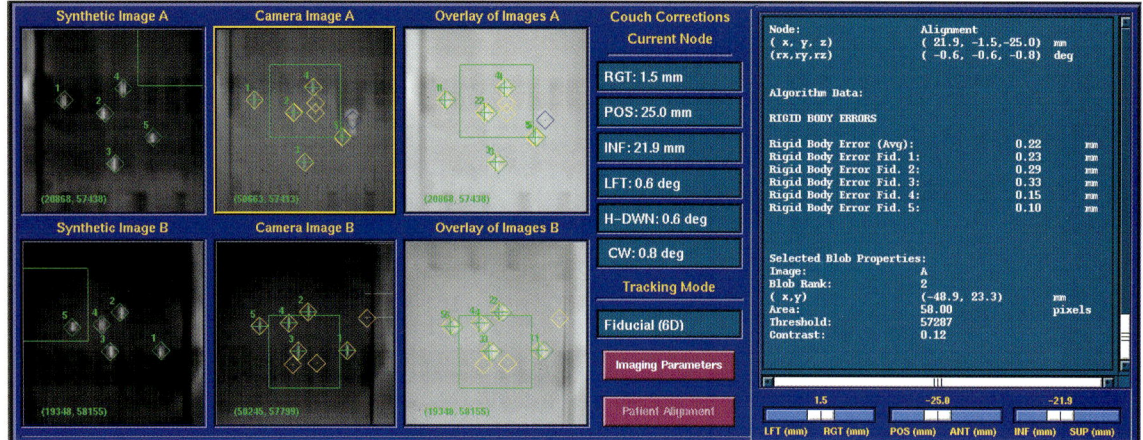

Figure 24. Blob characteristics of highlighted blob will be displayed in the Imaging Log

5. Rigid-body constraint errors:

Because accurate treatment delivery using fiducials requires that the fiducials remain fixed in relation to each other, the TLS is designed to check for cases of fiducial migration. When the location of an identified fiducial varies from the expected location by an amount greater than the "Rigid Body Distance Threshold" value specified in the *Imaging Parameters* menu, the TLS warns the operator with a *Fiducial Location Constraint Error* dialog box (Fig. 25). In this case, the fiducial that fails the rigid-body constraint will be marked in red, and the remaining fiducials will be marked in green (Fig. 26). Even though the remaining fiducials are correctly identified, no couch correction values can be returned because the entire configuration failed the extraction process due to the rigid-body error.

There are two ways in which a user can correct a rigid-body error. First, the fiducial that is causing the error may be incorrectly identified. If this is the case, the user can follow the steps in Section 4 above to encourage the TLS to identify the correct fiducial. If this fails or if the fiducial that caused the error was properly identified to begin with (indicating migration), the user should disable that fiducial in the "Use for Tracking" section of the *Tracking Parameters* menu.

In some cases, rigid-body errors can occur when patient position during treatment is not the same as

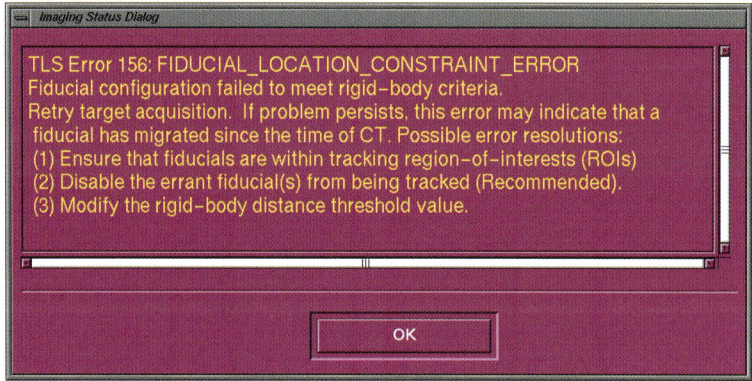

Figure 25. *Rigid-body Constraint Error* dialog box

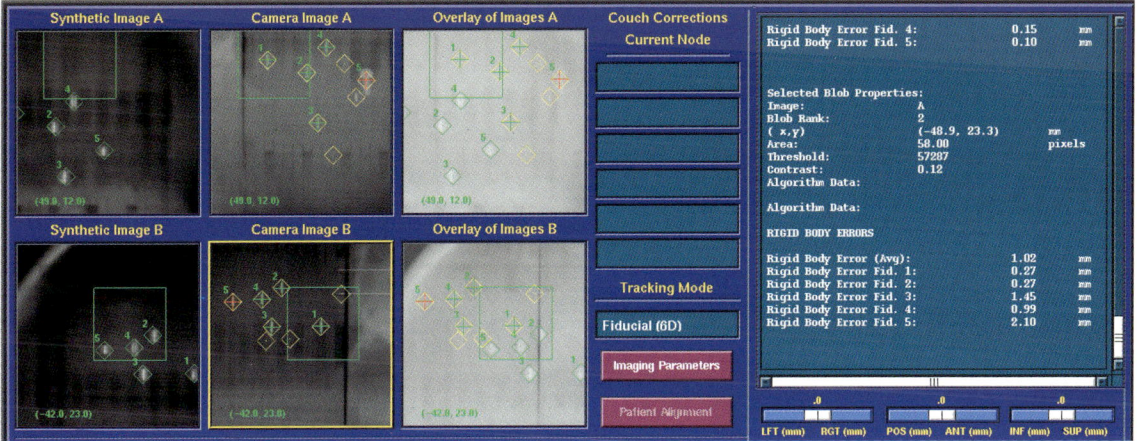

Figure 26. Rigid-body error showing the failed fiducial marked in red

the patient position in the planning CT. If it appears that the rigid-body error could be caused by changes in the alignment of the patient spine, repositioning the patient in the immobilization device may alleviate the error without adjustments to the *Tracking Parameters*.

6. Treatment delivery using fiducial tracking

Repositioning the patient in the Alignment mode is an iterative process. Once the patient has been moved into a position that is within the bounds of the *Imaging Parameters* and the physical limitations of the manipulator (1.0 cm translations in any direction), the "Start" button of the *Patient Alignment* window (Fig. 8) becomes active and the operator can commence treatment. However, individual cases may require that the patient be positioned more precisely than the outer limits of the treatment range. In these cases, the operator can progress through additional iterations of imaging and positioning until the translations and rotations have been minimized.

Once treatment commences, the system will automatically convert to Track mode, regardless of the mode used for alignment. During treatment delivery, extraction, correlation, and correction are all automated. If fiducials were properly identified during alignment, treatment delivery should proceed with few interruptions.

If a fiducial extraction error is encountered during treatment delivery, the *Fiducial Extraction Error* dialog box will appear and treatment will be interrupted. In such cases the user should progress through the dialog boxes back to the alignment screen. In most cases, acquisition of another image will result in proper fiducial extraction, and treatment can be started again. If fiducial extraction in the new image fails, check for redrawn ROIs. In cases where the ROI was drawn too tightly around the fiducial, small patient movements can cause the fiducial to move outside of the drawn ROI. Redrawing the ROI or restoring the default ROI will usually correct this situation.

In rare cases, treatment delivery can be interrupted repeatedly when a fiducial cannot be reliably tracked. If the fiducial cannot be consistently tracked after returning to the alignment screen multiple times, the user may wish to deactivate it for tracking to expedite the treatment process.

References

1. Kuduvalli, Gopinath; CyberKnife with DTS: Fiducials and Fiducial Tracking